# DOCUMENTATION MANUAL FOR

# WRITING SOAP NOTES

## IN OCCUPATIONAL THERAPY

# DOCUMENTATION MANUAL FOR

# WRITING SOAP NOTES

## IN OCCUPATIONAL THERAPY

*Sherry Borcherding, MA, OTR/L*
*University of Missouri*
*Columbia, Missouri*

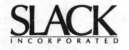

6900 Grove Road, Thorofare, New Jersey 08086

Publisher: John H. Bond
Editorial Director: Amy E. Drummond
Assistant Editor: Lauren Biddle Plummer

The work SLACK publishes is peer reviewed. Prior to publication, recognized leaders in the field, educators, and clinicians provide important feedback on the concepts and content that we publish. We welcome feedback on this work.

Borcherding, Sherry.
    Documentation manual for writing SOAP notes in occupational therapy/Sherry Borcherding.
        p. ; cm.
    Includes bibliographical references and index.
    ISBN 1-55642-441-8 (alk. paper)
    1. Occupational therapy--Practice. 2. Medical protocols. I. Title:Writing SOAP Notes in occupational therapy. II. Title.
    [DNLM: 1. Medical Records--Handbooks. 2. Occupational Therapy--methods--Handbooks. 3. Patient Care Planning--Handbooks. 4. Writing--Handbooks. WB 39 B726d 2000]
    RM735.4 .B67 2000
    615.8'2--dc21                                                    99-056947

Printed in Canada.

Published by:    SLACK Incorporated
                 6900 Grove Road
                 Thorofare, NJ 08086-9447 USA
                 Telephone: 856-848-1000
                 Fax: 856-853-5991
                 World Wide Web: http://www.slackinc.com

Contact SLACK Incorporated for more information about other books in this field or about the availability of our books from distributors outside the United States.

Last digit is print number: 10   9   8   7   6   5   4   3   2

# DEDICATION

This book is dedicated to the occupational therapy classes of 1998 and 1999 at the University of Missouri, who contributed their time and thoughts and allowed their notes to be used to teach others.

## Class of 1998

Jamie Allen
Michelle Boatman
Mary Bradshaw
Tammie Coon
Carie Copeland
Monica Davis
Jacquelyn Eder
Tara (Frazier) Grantham
Trisha Hall
Kristin Haskell
John Hettenhausen
Jason Hedrick
Paul Howard
Christina Howell
Terry Hudson
Adelle Hutchins
Mary Juergens
Katheryn Maddox
Karen Kitchen

Joy Le
Kristine Lottes
Ellen Niles
Theresa Parker
Cheryl Passanisi
Melody Peterson
Wynnette Phillips
Laura Pinnell
Jessi Saiter
Jennifer Stone
Rebecca Stranz
Marilyn Sunde
Durwood Tenny
Shelia M. Tenny
Kristen Todd
Brenda Watson
Rhonda Wolfe
Joanie Woodard
Heather Yamnitz

## Class of 1999

Kasiani Aslanidis
Nancy Belsly
Christy Boss
Bonnie Boyce
Madelon Butler
Ronda Christenson
Katie Conroy
Laurie Disharoon
Brenda Dunne
Nancy Ellis
Melissa Friederich
Brian Garrett
Gayla Gibson
Bridget Gunnels
Nicole Hays
Tracie Hope
Dawn Kelly
Victorya Korobov

Courtney Lockett
Desiree Mangone
Jennifer Meyer
Kim Neumann
Alyssia Niblett
Mariane Nicholls
Patricia Noonan
Laura Park
Rebecca Pohlmann
Paige Ridder
Susan Schmidt
Melanie Schoemehl
Jonalyn Siemer
Julie Smuckler
Kristen Stephenson
Stacy Stross
Erin Thomas
Dina Vatcha

# CONTENTS

# ACKNOWLEDGMENTS

Many people have contributed to the development of this manual. First, I would like to thank Diana Baldwin, Director of Occupational Therapy at the University of Missouri, for her patience in teaching me how to teach. Without her nurturing and support, I might have taken another pathway entirely. Thanks to Fred Dittrich for moving me as gracefully and quickly into the Information Age as I could tolerate. Thanks to Sandy Matsuda for editing the contributions, and for her loving friendship and support. Thanks to Doris O'Hara for bequeathing me the basic course material 7 years ago, and to Charlet Quay, Stephanie Owings, David Lackey, Lynne White, and LeaAnn Brittain for filling in the gaps in my knowledge base. Thanks to Leanna Garrison for being the Format Goddess. Thanks to Lenore Ball, Theresa Lackey, Chris Nelson, Linda Eagle, and Randy Kilgrore for their help and support. But most of all, I would like to thank the students who have taught me so much about documentation over the past 7 years.

# ABOUT THE AUTHOR

Sherry Borcherding currently serves as a faculty member at University of Missouri-Columbia, a Research I University, where she has taught for 7 years. She teaches disability awareness, loss and grief, and a three-semester fieldwork sequence designed to develop critical thinking, clinical reasoning, and documentation skills. She has also taught clinical ethics, frames of reference, psychopathology, long-term care, and wellness. Two of her courses are designated as campus writing courses, and one is credentialed for computer and information proficiency. Sherry is frequently invited to present on collaborative learning and peer review as teaching strategies. In addition, she was one of a small group of campus faculty initially selected to develop web-based courses.

Sherry graduated with honors from Texas Women's University with a BS in occupational therapy and went on to complete her masters in special education at George Peabody College in Nashville, TN. Following her staff positions in rehabilitation, home health, and pediatrics, she assumed a number of management roles including Chief Occupational Therapist at East Texas Treatment Center, Director of Occupational Therapy at Mid-Missouri Mental Health Center, and Director of Rehabilitation Services at Transitional Housing Agency. She has also planned, designed, and directed occupational therapy programs at Charles E. Still Hospital in Jefferson City, MO and at Charter Behavioral Health Center in Columbia, MO.

Besides teaching, Sherry consults on quality assurance issues for local behavioral health centers and has a private practice devoted to complementary and alternative therapies. She is certified in CranioSacral Therapy at the techniques level through Upledger Institute and is attuned as a Reiki Master. For leisure, Sherry enjoys folk dance, music, and all kinds of three-dimensional art. Her pottery has appeared in three local shows over the past 4 years.

# CHAPTER 1
## Documenting the Treatment Process in Occupational Therapy

## Introduction

Welcome to a new style of writing. The first time you see an experienced occupational therapist write a treatment note in a patient's chart you might be tempted to think you will never be able to do it yourself. Just the technical language alone can be intimidating, and then there is the amazing attention to detail in the patient observation, the insightful assessment, and the plan that just seems to roll off her pen while you are wondering how long it will take you to be able to predict a course of treatment like that. Professional documentation is a skill, and like any skill, it can be learned. Learning a skill, whether it is downhill skiing, playing the violin, or composing a treatment note, requires two things of you: 1) Instruction on how to do it—what to put into each section of the note, and 2) Practice—with feedback on which parts are correct and which still need work. This manual is designed to get you started with both parts of the process. Information is provided on each part of the documentation process, and the worksheets are designed to let you practice each step as you learn it.

The format for writing SOAP notes provided in this manual is one that is reimbursable under both Medicare Part B and managed care. While all notes do not have to meet these requirements, the Medicare B and managed care standards are the most rigorous. If you learn to meet these standards you are not likely to be denied by any third party payer.

Current occupational therapy practice is in many ways determined by which services are reimbursable, and documentation of patient care is the vehicle by which that service is communicated. Many therapists were not taught how to write effective notes and had to learn it on the job. They have learned what works in their own situation, but may or may not be prepared to meet the requirements of other settings.

In the *Standards for an Accredited Educational Program for the Occupational Therapist* (Accreditation Council for Occupational Therapy Education [ACOTE], 1998a) and the *Standards for an Accredited Educational Program for the Occupational Therapy Assistant* (ACOTE, 1998b) for educational programs, we learn that coursework must provide competency in being able to "document occupational therapy services to ensure accountability of service provision and to meet standards for reimbursement of services. Documentation shall effectively communicate the need and rationale for occupational therapy services" (ACOTE, 1998a, Section B.4.10; ACOTE, 1998b, Section B.3.4). This manual will provide you with a mechanism for becoming competent in documentation skills.

The content of this manual reflects the scope of our practice and emphasizes the basis of our services, e.g., the use of occupation through occupational performance. Material from four official documents of the American Occupational Therapy Association (AOTA) has been incorporated:

- *Elements of Clinical Documentation* (AOTA, 1998a)
- *Uniform Terminology for Occupational Therapy*, Third Edition (AOTA, 1998d)
- *The Guide to Occupational Therapy Practice* (Moyers, 1999)
- *Standards of Practice for Occupational Therapy* (AOTA, 1998c)

Although occupational therapists write in more than one format, this manual presents a systematic approach to writing one form of documentation, the SOAP note. The manual is designed as a teaching tool and is most effective if used as a workbook, reading the information in each section, completing each exercise, then checking your answers against the suggested answers. The material presented here grew out of a course on documentation that has been taught for 7 years for seniors at the University of Missouri, Columbia, a Carnegie Research I University. It has been field-tested to be sure it is understandable and effective in helping you learn both documentation and clinical reasoning.

The information in this manual has been arranged in the order that it is most easily learned, with the more straightforward concepts being offered first. More complex concepts build on these as clinical reasoning is developed. *Chapter 2: The Medical Record* provides an introduction to the medical record—its function, uses, and history. The history of the SOAP note is included, along with the mechanics of writing in the record. Also included in Chapter 2 is a list of standard abbreviations to be used in completing the exercises in the manual.

*Chapter 3: Writing Functional Problem Statements* discusses the mechanics of writing problem statements. After you evaluate a patient, you develop a problem list, which is essentially a list of those areas of occupational performance that you think you can positively impact during treatment. From this list, you formulate **functional problem statements**. After the problems have been defined and prioritized, goals are formulated with the patient. The goals are worded in behavioral and measurable terms. This includes both long-term goals (**goals**) and short term goals (**objectives**). *Chapter 4: Writing Functional and Measurable Goals and Objectives* discusses the format for writing goals and objectives. Worksheets are provided for practice, and some examples of well-written problem and goal statements offer you some help if you are having trouble.

The next four chapters teach the four sections of the SOAP format (**Subjective, Objective, Assessment, and Plan**), that has been introduced and explained in Chapter 2. Multiple examples are presented for each section, and worksheets are provided for practice. It is difficult to learn documentation without observing treatment sessions upon which to base the notes, and it is assumed that you will have access to a treatment setting in which to document. Following the chapters that teach basic skills, treatment planning is discussed in *Chapter 9: Treatment Planning*, since the treatment plan is a vital part of the initial evaluation.

*Chapter 10: Documenting Different Stages of Treatment* discusses the different kinds of notes that are written at different stages of the treatment process. From the first notation in the chart that a referral has been received to the closing lines of the discharge summary, registered occupational therapists and certified occupational therapy assistants document the many and varied activities of the treatment process. The specific content of the note, the format of the note, and the time lines required vary according to type of setting, accrediting agencies involved, and requirements of third party payers. The contents required for each type of note are described in *Elements of Clinical Documentation* (Revision) (AOTA, 1998a). **Intake notes** are brief entries acknowledging orders received either in writing or by telephone. Intake notes are not always required and are not addressed in this manual. We will address the requirements for the following kinds of notes.

### Initial Evaluation Reports

Before beginning treatment, the occupational therapist evaluates the patient to determine whether occupational therapy is appropriate for this patient, and if so, what kind of treatment will be most useful. Each setting has its own way of evaluating a patient. A mental health center, for example, may not do the same kind of initial evaluation as a public school or skilled nursing facility. Initial evaluations are usually documented on forms provided by the setting, but may also be done in a SOAP format.

### Treatment, Contact, or Visit Notes

Each time treatment is provided by the occupational therapist, notation is made of what occurred during the treatment session. In some settings, each session is documented using a contact note (also called a treatment note or visit note). In other settings, the therapist makes notes to use later in writing progress notes, but no formalized visit note is required. Many different formats are used for writing contact notes, but in this manual the SOAP format will be taught.

### Progress Notes

At the end of a specified period of time, a progress note is written explaining how the patient is responding to treatment and detailing any changes to be made in the treatment plan. Some settings, such as mental health centers, require weekly progress notes. Others, such as residential facilities, require monthly notes. Other settings may use different time periods for reporting. Progress notes may also be written in different formats, but will be taught in a SOAP format in this manual.

### Reevaluation Notes

The reevaluation that is part of the occupational therapy treatment process may be documented in a formal reevaluation report in some settings. For example, in a managed care setting, a patient may need to be reevaluated in order to be recertified for treatment after the number of visits initially allocated are completed.

### Discharge Notes

At the end of treatment, a discharge note is written detailing the course of treatment, the accomplishment (or not) of goals, the status at the time of discharge, any home program that may have been recommended, and any other recommendations or referrals. Some settings provide a specific form for the discharge note and other facilities may use the same form that was used for the evaluation. Others use a different format. For purposes of this manual, a SOAP format will be used.

*Chapter 11: Documentation in Different Practice Settings* discusses the special requirements of different kinds of practice settings (mental health, long-term care, school-based practice, and consultation), and *Chapter 12: Making Good Notes Even Better* is a review of what you have learned. Notes from a variety of treatment settings are provided at the end of the manual in *Chapter 13: Examples of Different Kinds of Notes*, in addition to the examples scattered throughout the book. *Appendix: Suggestions for Completing the Worksheets* provides "answers" for the worksheets. However, since there are many "right" ways to answer, these must be viewed as suggestions rather than the only correct answers.

# Skilled Occupational Therapy

Throughout this manual occupational therapy service is described as skilled occupational therapy. This term was coined in Medicare regulations which define the difference between skilled and non-skilled services. Since Medicare Part B requirements are being followed in this manual to insure that your services will not be denied payment, it is important to know that Medicare reimburses those interventions that are identified as skilled and does **not** reimburse those considered non-skilled. **Skilled** services are those that require decision-making and highly complex competencies and that have a well-defined knowledge base of human functioning and occupational performance. **Nonskilled** services are defined as those that are routine or maintenance type of therapy, both of which could be carried out by nonprofessional personnel or caregivers. The use of "skilled" in this manual emphasizes the necessity of documenting your occupational therapy interventions clearly as those activities requiring the services of a qualified registered occupational therapist or a certified occupational therapy assistant (Lopes, 1998).

# Uniform Terminology

Before we discuss documenting the treatment process, we need to differentiate skilled occupational therapy from other disciplines in the health professions. As occupational therapists, we treat people who have problems in areas of **occupational performance**. This is important to note, because this is what we will document. The practice of occupational therapy can be divided into **performance areas** (activities of daily living, work, and leisure) and **performance components** (the underlying sensory, motor, cognitive, and psychological factors necessary to be independent or successful in the performance areas). In documenting occupational therapy services, the focus on performance **areas** is critical for showing the necessity for skilled occupational therapy and preventing any question of duplication of services. Skilled occupational therapy may be required to treat functional losses in the following areas.

## Activities of Daily Living

There are several levels of activities of daily living, and all of these fall within the scope of skilled occupational therapy. **Basic** activities of daily living (ADL) are tasks that are necessary for self-care and personal independence, such as bathing, grooming, hygiene, dressing, eating, toileting, communication, and functional mobility. **Instrumental** activities of daily living (IADL) require more complex problem-solving and social skills and include such tasks as money management, cleaning, laundry, child care, driving, shopping, and meal preparation. Therapists who work with persons with brain injury also talk about executive functions, which are lost in frontal lobe damage. The executive functions include such activities as planning, goal setting, and organizational tasks. In documenting services, it is necessary to demonstrate why a skilled therapist is needed to perform the task, rather than a family member, aide, or physical therapist (Pedretti, 1996).

In a mental health setting, you would want to consider not just the physical ability to care for self and to interact with the community, but also the emotional components that might be limiting performance. Rather than being limited by a physical factor, a patient with mental illness might be limited by motivation or by the absence of adequate social skills. In a school setting, the ADL tasks of the child are those that allow him to be successful in school, such as the ability to sit still in a chair, hold a pencil, or form letters on a piece of paper.

## Work

For younger people, the ability to return to work may be the primary focus of skilled occupational therapy treatment rather than the ability to care for oneself. Whereas Medicare is interested in a person more than 65 years of age being able to perform self-care tasks, workman's compensation is interested in a person less than 65 years being able to return to work. It is important to consider your payment source as well as your patient's interests and priorities when selecting the treatment goals and interventions you plan to use.

## Leisure

Those activities that are neither work nor self-care often fall into the category of leisure. Particularly for older people, leisure is a very important part of occupational performance, and yet the limitations of some payment sources may make it a difficult area to document. Often leisure activities are treated by working on the performance components needed for doing the task, rather than approaching the task directly.

## Performance Components

Performance components that limit occupational performance also fall within the scope of skilled occupational therapy, as long as there is documentation that a change in the performance component will result in a change in some area of occupational performance. Functional limitations might include such areas as lack of sensory awareness, impaired strength or range of motion, uncoordination, abnormal muscle tone, impaired body schema, perceptual deficits, impaired balance or mobility, delusions, disturbances of mood and thought, and environmental barriers. In documenting a treatment session devoted to improving one of these underlying factors, it is critical to tie it to the function that is expected to improve because of the treatment. It is also critical to document in some way that the skill of a registered occupational therapist was needed to accomplish the task.

## Safety Concerns

The ability to perform a task must include the ability to do it safely. Safety concerns such as a high probability of falling, lack of environmental awareness, severe pain (either physical or emotional), the lack of skin sensation, abnormally aggressive or destructive behaviors, or suicide risk all fall within the scope of skilled occupational therapy. Safety is usually seen by third party payers, such as Medicare, as a cost-effective service because it prevents costly further injury.

## Prevention of Secondary Complications

Treatment focused on prevention is within the scope of skilled occupational therapy if it can be shown that the patient has a high risk of developing these complications. These might include prevention of progressive joint contractures, fracture non-union, and skin breakdown, as well as instruction in joint protection and energy conservation.

# Roles of the Registered Occupational Therapist and Certified Occupational Therapy Assistant

The registered occupational therapist and the certified occupational therapy assistant have different roles and responsibilities in documenting the occupational therapy treatment process. The AOTA (1998c) provides guidelines in the *Standards of Practice for Occupational Therapy* for the types of responsibility for different personnel. These guidelines are considered "best practice" but they may differ from state and federal laws that delineate mandatory documentation requirements. Sometimes reimbursement organizations specify who would be an approved documenter for reimbursement purposes. You as a therapist are accountable for adhering to the mandatory policies and procedures adopted by state and federal regulatory agencies, but you will find the standards established by AOTA useful in interpreting and following regulations.

The role of the certified occupational therapy assistant is described in the *Standards of Practice for Occupational Therapy* (AOTA, 1998c) Sections IV.6, V.1. & 2., VI.4., and VII.4., as one of contributing to the data in the initial evaluation, treatment plan, reevaluation and discharge note under the supervision of the registered occupational therapist and concurring with relevant laws and regulations. The certified occupational therapy assistant may document the patient's progress and response during treatment implementation within regulatory limitations.

# Conclusion

In the following pages you will be introduced to the medical record and to the ins-and-outs of your documentation in the record. There will be ample explanation and practice so that in the end **you** will be the occupational therapist we talked about in the beginning paragraph whose documentation was so amazing to the beginning student.

# CHAPTER 2
## The Medical Record

## Definition and Purpose

The medical record is "a compilation of pertinent facts of a patient's life and health history, including past and present illness(es) and treatment(s) written by the health professionals contributing to that patient's care" (Huffman, 1994, p. 28). Like so many other aspects of health care, the medical record is undergoing vast changes as we move further into the information age. The purpose of the record is documentation of the patient's illness and treatment, particularly the current episode. Although the medical record is the physical property of the facility that compiles it, the information contained in the record is actually the property of the patient, and that information must be made available to the patient or to his legal representative upon appropriate request (Huffman, 1994).

## History

Health care can be traced back approximately 7,000 years to early medicine men who were thought to be able to communicate with the spirit world. Written records can be found as early as 2700 BC in Egypt (Abdelhak, Grostick, Haniken, & Jacobs, 1996). After one of the first hospitals in America was incorporated in Pennsylvania in 1792, its secretary, Benjamin Franklin, began to keep records of patients' names, addresses, disorders, and dates of admission and discharge. These early records were often kept in ledgers, and were brief and handwritten. As medicine advanced, so did the complexity and detail of the medical record. A profession (now called Health Information Management) was created to oversee the record. Most hospitals today are moving toward a computerized record, with a vision that someday paper will no longer be necessary.

## The Problem-Oriented Medical Record

In the 1960s a physician named Lawrence Weed decided to reorganize the way medical records were kept (Huffman, 1994). He saw the medical record as being arranged for the convenience of the staff, rather than ordered for the highest good of the patient. He developed what he called the Problem-Oriented Medical Record (POMR), which was designed to be a patient-centered method of recording. He wanted to see the record organized into four sections:

1. A database, containing the history and physical, evaluations by all disciplines, lab results, etc.
2. A list of the patient's problems.
3. An interdisciplinary treatment plan, developed by all the staff working with the patient.
4. Progress notes written in chronological order, regardless of discipline.

By organizing the chart in this manner, all information on any of the presenting problems is in one area, easy to find. You don't have to search the chart to see what each discipline has to say about that area of concern. The progress notes are also consolidated rather than being organized by discipline, so that all the information regarding what has happened for/to the patient on that day is in one place. In this way, it is easy for any of the medical staff to read progress notes for the last 24 hours and know everything that is current without having to search several sections of the chart for the necessary information.

As a part of the more patient-centered approach to documentation, Weed recommended that the progress note be organized into four sections including the patient's own perception of the situation, which had heretofore been considered irrelevant. These four sections included:

- **S (Subjective)**: the patient's perception of the treatment being received, the progress, limitations, needs, and problems. Normally the subjective section of the note is brief. In an initial evaluation note, however, the "S" might be longer, since it will contain the information you obtained in your interview.
- **(Objective)**: the health professional's observations of the treatment being provided. In an evaluation note, this section also contains of all the measurable, quantifiable, and observable data that was collected. In an initial assessment, the first two sections form the database from which a problem list and treatment plan evolve. Some facilities have combined the first two sections into a composite category called **data**, and have adapted Weed's SOAP notes into DAP notes. For purposes of this manual, we will continue to use the two discrete sections.
- **A (Assessment)**: the health professional's interpretation of the meaning of the events reported in the Objective section. This section includes functional limitations, along with your expectations of the patient's ability to benefit from therapy (sometimes called rehabilitation potential). An initial evaluation also contains the problem list that is one of the key elements of the POMR method of charting. In a progress note, the assessment component contains an explicit statement of progress or the lack of progress. In a problem-oriented record, each progress note is tied to a problem from the patient's problem list. That problem is noted at the beginning of the note.
- **P (Plan)**: what the health professional plans to do next to continue with the goals and objectives in the treatment plan. In an initial evaluation, this section contains the treatment plan along with the anticipated frequency and duration of treatment.

For almost 30 years Weed's system was popular in hospitals and rehabilitation centers. Gradually, however, facilities have returned to a more source-oriented medical record, containing sections for each discipline. Even so, the SOAP format of progress notes has remained popular in facilities that no longer use the POMR.

Remember that SOAP is just a format—an outline for organizing information. Any note can be written in this format, although some notes lend themselves to it better than others. For example, you could write an initial assessment in a SOAP format, or a discharge summary, or a daily note, as well as a progress note. An initial assessment, however, can be quite lengthy when written this way, as it will contain a history, summary of functional problems, short- and long-term goals, prior level of functioning, and the beginning treatment plan. For this reason, most practice settings would not use a SOAP format for the initial evaluation report, even if that facility used SOAP for its treatment and progress notes.

The SOAP format is an alternative to narrative notes, which tend to be disorganized and subjective. It forces the writer to look at all four aspects of the treatment session, and to present the information contained in the note in an orderly fashion. A more detailed discussion of each section of the note follows in Chapters 5 through 8.

# Users and Uses of the Medical Record

The medical record is a communication tool, and has many uses and many different users. It is important to consider all your different audiences when you make an entry in the patient's record.

## Patient Care Management

The record is one of the ways the treatment team communicates with each other about the day to day aspects of a patient's care. Other therapists in your own department or members of the treatment team will read your notes in order to coordinate care. In your note you share the results of your evaluation, report your patient's progress toward the goals, and advise other members of the team of your plan for continuing care, all of which are important to the treatment team. In a situation where occupational therapy is provided 7 days per week, one occupational therapist may not be providing all of the patient's care and may depend upon the treatment notes to find out what treatment was provided in her absence.

## Reimbursement

The medical record is the source document for what services were provided, and for what services may be billed. It is used in billing to substantiate reimbursement claims. For example, if there were a question about the duration and frequency provided, the record would be the source document used to answer that question.

## The Legal System

The medical record is a legal document that substantiates what occurred during a patient's illness/treatment. If you as an occupational therapist have to appear in court to testify, you will be very glad that your documentation is clear and thorough. Sometimes court cases occur years after the event or treatment that is being contested. You may not even remember the event or the patient. What you have written in the medical record will provide you with the information you need in order to testify.

## Quality Improvement

Most facilities have a Quality Improvement (QI) Committee whose duty it is to oversee the adequacy and appropriateness of the care that is being provided. This committee is in charge of finding and solving problems in patient care. The medical record is one of the primary sources of information used in the QI process.

## Research

The record is also used to provide data for medical research. Some research uses individual data specific to that patient while other research uses aggregate data where no patient name is attached to the data. In either case, the source document is often the medical record.

## Accreditation

Accrediting agencies such as the Joint Commission for the Accreditation of Health Care Organizations (JCAHO) and the Commission on Accreditation of Rehabilitation Facilities (CARF) review your notes to ascertain whether the extent and quality of services provided by your facility and/or your department meet the standards of care set by the accrediting agency. If your facility is found to not be in compliance, accreditation may be withdrawn. For example the Health Care Finance Administration (HCFA) accredits facilities that bill for Medicare. If the facility does not meet HCFA standards, all claims made by that facility for Medicare services would be denied. The medical record is one of the primary sources of information used during an accreditation visit.

## Education

The record may be used as a teaching tool. A student uses the medical record to gain information about patients, and about quality and appropriate occupational therapy treatment.

## Public Health

The record is also used to identify and to document the incidence of certain diseases, such as tuberculosis or HIV.

## Utilization Management

In a hospital setting, the Utilization Review Committee is charged with determining how services in the facility are being utilized. For example, the committee may want to know what kinds of patients are being seen and what kind of care is being provided, and whether these are appropriate to the mission of the facility.

## Business Development

Management teams use the information contained in the record to plan and market the services provided by the facility. For example, the director may want to know whether or not there are enough cases of eating disorders being admitted to open a special eating disorders unit.

## The Patient

Another significant user is the patient himself. When you are writing in the medical record, always remember that the patient owns the information in his own record and may choose to exercise his right to read what you have written.

# Writing in the Record

Since the medical record is not only a communication tool during the patient's hospital stay, but also the source document for financial, legal, and clinical accountability, the record should show the following:

- What services you provided and when
- What happened and what was said
- How the client responded to the service provided
- Why your skill as an OT was needed rather than the services of an aide or family member

Before you write anything in the medical record, make these assumptions:

- Someone else will have to read and understand what I write because I may be out sick or out of town the next time this patient needs to be treated.
- The entry I am about to make will be the one scrutinized by an HCFA review team or a Blue Cross representative. If I were a funding source, would I want to pay for the services I am about to record?
- My patient will exercise his right to read this record.

It is critical to know your payment sources when documenting. Some payers are looking for quite different outcomes than others. With a Medicare patient, you will discuss activities of daily living and write goals for self care activities. With a workers' compensation case, you will write goals that are oriented to return to work. With home care, you may need to document that your patient is unable to leave home to receive services or that education on safety issues was provided to the caregiver. With a child, you will need to focus on developmental needs or educationally related services identified in the Individualized Education Plan (IEP).

Also remember these facts when planning to write in a patient's record:

- Accuracy is your best protection against problems. You cannot be accurate if you wait too long to record what happened.
- A note in the patient's chart is going to be a reflection of your professional identity and abilities, as well as a reflection of your department and OT as a profession.
- No activity or contact is ever considered a service that has been provided until a clinical entry is in the record. In terms of fiscal and legal accountability, "If it isn't written, it didn't happen."

Helpful hints on writing notes:

- Be as concise as possible without leaving out pertinent data.
- Avoid generalities.
- Report behavior and avoid judgments except in the assessment portion of your data.
- Be sparse with technical jargon that may be unfamiliar to the reader.

# The Mechanics of Documentation

There are a few rules that must be followed when writing in the medical record:

1. **Always use waterproof black ink.**
   After a certain period of time medical records are microfilmed, and black ink is the only color that microfilms adequately.
2. **Never use correction fluid.**
   Using white out in a medical record is considered illegally altering the record. The medical record is a legal document that must stand as originally written.

3. **Correct errors.**
   If you make an error in the medical record, draw one line through it, write your correction, and initial the change.

   _Pt. able to dress lower body with_ ~~verbal cues~~ <sup>S𝔅</sup> _min_ Ⓐ _using a reacher._

   In a problem oriented medical chart, if you inadvertently write your note in the wrong patient's chart, draw a single line through the entire entry and write "wrong chart" beside it with your signature.

   If you need to add something after you have written and signed your note, write an addendum with the current date and time.

4. **Be sure all required data is present.**
   _The Elements of Clinical Documentation_ (Revision) (AOTA, 1998a) and _The Guide to Occupational Therapy Practice_ (Moyers, 1999) specify the contents for each type of note you may be writing. This information will be covered in Chapter 10. Make certain that your note contains all the necessary information, and remember, it is absolutely critical that you sign and date your note.

5. **Be concise.**
   In today's health care system, busy professionals are often pressed for time and appreciate being able to read what you have written in the shortest time possible. Your own time for documentation will also be limited under today's productivity standards.

6. **Use appropriate terminology for the recipients of services.**
   When referring to the people who use occupational therapy services, we have traditionally referred to them as patients or clients based on the setting where services were received. However, as practice areas are rapidly changing and expanding, the AOTA has addressed the use of terminology in the official document _Service Delivery in Occupational Therapy_ (AOTA, 1998b) as follows:

   > Service provision occurs directly with individual, groups, programs, or organizations. Depending on the setting in which the occupational therapy practitioner works, various terms may be used for individual client (e.g., patient, consumer, resident, participant, student, teacher, employer, or administrator). Group clients may include families, teams, or others with common needs. (p. 100)

   For the purposes of this manual, names have been fabricated to protect the privacy of those people who receive our services. The terms patient, consumer, client, resident, individual, and veteran, as well as first names have been used. In a note that says "Mr. P. was seen in his home..." please understand that he is being called "Mr. P." for purposes of confidentiality. In your note, you would use his whole name.

7. **Use abbreviations.**
   Use **only** the abbreviations that are approved by your facility. While it saves time to use symbols and abbreviations, remember that your notes may be read by someone with a high school education who knows little about occupational therapy and who will determine whether or not to pay for your services. It is wise to be sure that the person is able to understand what you have written. Your facility will be able to furnish a list of the abbreviations it allows so the abbreviations and symbols you use will be validated if there is a question. **Do not** make up your own abbreviations, and do not use any abbreviation that is not on your facility's approved list. Remember, it is **permitted** to use abbreviations, but it is not necessary. You are permitted to write out any word instead of shortening it. In this manual you will find that some notes use more abbreviations and symbols than others (Table 2-1).

# Table 2-1
## Abbreviations and Symbols

| Abbreviation | Meaning | Abbreviation | Meaning | Abbreviation | Meaning |
|---|---|---|---|---|---|
| A | anterior; assessment | CAT | computerized axial tomography | EOB | edge of bed |
| Ⓐ | assistance | | | ER | emergency room |
| ā | before | CBC | complete blood count | ETOH | ethyl alcohol |
| AAROM | active assistive range of motion | cc | cubic centimeter | eval. | evaluation |
| | | CC | chief complaint | ext. | extension |
| ABI | acquired brain injury | CCU | coronary (cardiac) care unit | F | Fahrenheit; Fair (muscle strength grade of 3) |
| a.c. | before meals | | | | |
| abd | abduction | CGA | contact guard assist | f | female |
| ACTH | adrenocorticotrophic hormone | CHF | congestive heart failure | F.A.C.P. | fellow of the American College of Physicians |
| | | CHI | closed head injury | | |
| add | adduction | cm | centimeter | F.A.C.S. | fellow of the American College of Surgeons |
| ADD | Attention Deficit Disorder | CNS | central nervous system | | |
| ADHD | Attention Deficit Hyperactivity Disorder | $CO_2$ | carbon dioxide | FBS | fasting blood sugar |
| | | c/o | complains of | FH | family history |
| ADL | activity of daily living | cont. | continue | flex. | flexion |
| ad lib. | as desired | cmc | carpometacarpal | fl oz | fluid ounce |
| AIDS | acquired immunodeficiency syndrome | COPD | chronic obstructive pulmonary disease | FROM | functional range of motion |
| AE | above elbow | COTA | certified occupational therapy assistant | FSH | follicle-stimulating hormone |
| AK | above knee | | | | |
| AKA | above knee amputation | CP | cerebral palsy | ft. | foot, feet (the measurement, not the body part) |
| am, AM | morning | CPR | cardiopulmonary resuscitation | | |
| AMA | against medical advice | | | FUO | fever, unknown origin |
| AMB | ambulation | CSF | cerebrospinal fluid | FWB | full weight bearing |
| amt | amount | CT | computed tomography | Fx | fracture |
| AP | anterior-posterior | CTR | carpal tunnel release | G | Good (muscle strength grade of 4) |
| AROM | active range of motion | cu mm | cubic millimeter | | |
| ASA | aspirin | CVA | cerebrovascular accident | GB | gallbladder |
| ASAP | as soon as possible | CXR | chest x-ray | GI | gastrointestinal |
| ASHD | arteriosclerotic heart disease | d | day | gm | gram |
| | | Ⓓ | dependent | g, gr | grain |
| ASIS | anterior superior iliac spine | D&C | dilation and curettage | GTT | glucose tolerance test |
| | | DC, D/C | discharge; discontinue | GYN | gynecology |
| Ⓑ | bilateral | D.C. | doctor of chiropractic medicine | h | hour |
| BE | below elbow | | | HA, H/A | headache |
| b.i.d. | twice a day | D.D.S. | doctor of dental surgery | H&P | history and physical |
| BK | below knee | DIP | distal interphalangeal joint | HBV | hepatitis B virus |
| BKA | below knee amputation | | | HCT, Hct | hematocrit |
| BM | black male; bowel movement | DJD | degenerative joint disease | HEENT | head, eyes, ears, nose, throat |
| BP | blood pressure | DLS | daily living skills | HEP | home exercise program |
| BRP | bathroom privileges | D.O. | doctor of osteopathic medicine | HGB, Hgb | hemoglobin |
| BS | blood sugar | | | HIV | human immunodeficiency virus |
| B/S | bedside | DM | diabetes mellitus | | |
| BUN | blood urea nitrogen | dr | dram | HOB | head of bed |
| Bx | biopsy | Dr. | doctor | HRT | hormone replacement therapy |
| c̄ | with | DTR | deep tendon reflex | | |
| C | Celsius; centigrade | DVT | deep vein thrombosis | HR | heart rate |
| CA | carcinoma; cancer | Dx | diagnosis | hr. | hour |
| C&S | culture and sensitivity | ECG | electrocardiogram | hs | at bedtime |
| CABG | coronary artery bypass graft | ECHO | echocardiogram | Ht | height |
| | | EEG | electroencephalogram | HTN | hypertension |
| CAD | coronary artery disease | EKG | electrocardiogram | Hx | history |
| cal | calories | EMG | electromyogram | Ⓘ | independent |
| cap | capsule | ENT | ear, nose, throat | | |

# Table 2-1 (continued)
## Abbreviations and Symbols

| | | | | | |
|---|---|---|---|---|---|
| IADL | instrumental activity of daily living | O₂ | oxygen | PTA | physical therapist assistant; prior to admission |
| ICU | intensive care unit | OX4 | oriented to time, place, person, situation | PTCA | percutaneous transluminal coronary angioplasty |
| IDDM | insulin-dependent diabetes mellitus | OB | obstetrics | | |
| | | OBS | organic brain syndrome | | |
| IM | intramuscular | OH | occupational history | PTH | parathyroid hormone |
| IMP | impression | OP | outpatient | PWB | partial weight bearing |
| in. | inches | OR | operating room | Px | physical examination |
| IP | inpatient | ORIF | open reduction, internal fixation | q | every |
| IUD | intrauterine device | | | qd | every day |
| IV | intravenous | OT | occupational therapist; occupational therapy | qh | every hour |
| kg | kilogram | | | q2h | every two hours |
| KUB | kidney, ureter, bladder | oz | ounce | q.i.d. | four times a day |
| L | left; liter | p̄ | after | qn | every night |
| Ⓛ | left | P | plan; posterior; pulse; Poor (muscle strength grade of 2) | q.o.d. | every other day |
| lb | pound | | | qt. | quart |
| LE | lower extremity | | | R | right; respiration |
| LLQ | left lower quadrant | PA | posterior anterior; physician's assistant | Ⓡ | right |
| LP | lumbar puncture | | | RA | rheumatoid arthritis |
| LTG | long-term goal | PAP | Papanicolaou test (smear) | RBC | red blood cell count |
| LUQ | left upper quadrant | PDD | Pervasive Developmental Disorder | R.D. | registered dietician |
| m | murmur; meter; male | | | re: | regarding |
| max | maximum | PE | physical examination | rehab | rehabilitation |
| Meds. | medications | per | by | resp | respiratory; respiration |
| MFT | muscle function test | PET | positron emission tomography | RLQ | right lower quadrant |
| MD | muscular dystrophy; medical doctor | | | R/O | rule out |
| | | PFT | pulmonary function testing | ROM | range of motion |
| mg | milligram | | | ROS | review of symptoms |
| MI | myocardial infarction | Ph.D. | doctor of philosophy | RROM | resistive range of motion |
| ml | milliliter | PID | pelvic inflammatory disease | R.T. | respiratory therapist; recreation therapist |
| min | minutes; minimum | | | | |
| mm | millimeter | PIH | pregnancy induced hypertension | RTC | return to clinic |
| mo. | month | | | RTO | return to office |
| mod | moderate | PIP | proximal interphalangeal | RUQ | right upper quadrant |
| MP, MCP | metacarpophalangeal | p.m., PM | afternoon | RSD | reflex sympathetic dystrophy |
| MRI | magnetic resonance imaging | PMH | past medical history | | |
| | | PNF | proprioceptive neuromuscular facilitation | Rx | recipe; Latin *take thou* prescription |
| MS | multiple sclerosis; musculoskeletal | PNI | peripheral nerve injury | s̄ | without |
| MSH | melanocyte-stimulating hormone | PNS | peripheral nervous system | S | subjective |
| | | | | SBA | stand by assistance |
| MVP | mitral valve prolapse | p.o. | by mouth | SH | social history |
| N | Normal (muscle strength grade of 5) | POMR | problem-oriented medical record | Sig: | instruction to patient |
| | | | | SLE | systemic lupus erythematosus |
| NDT | neurodevelopmental treatment | pos. | positive | SOC | start of care |
| neg. | negative | poss | possible | SOAP | subjective objective assessment plan |
| NG | nasogastric | post op | post operation | | |
| NKA | no known allergy | pre op | pre operation | SOB | shortness of breath |
| NKDA | no known drug allergy | p.r.n. | as needed | SNF | skilled nursing facility |
| noc. | night | pro | pronation | SpGr | specific gravity |
| NPO | nothing by mouth | PROM | passive range of motion | S/P | status post |
| NSR | normal sinus rhythm | pt. | patient | sq | subcutaneous |
| NWB | non-weightbearing | PT | physical therapist, physical therapy | SR | systems review |
| O | objective; oriented | | | STAT | immediately |

# Table 2-1 (continued)
## Abbreviations and Symbols

| | | | | | |
|---|---|---|---|---|---|
| STD | sexually transmitted disease | TSH | thyroid-stimulating hormone | ♀ | female |
| STG | short-term goal | Tx | treatment; traction | ↓ | down; downward; decrease |
| suppos | suppository | UA | urinalysis | ↑ | up; upward; increase |
| sup | supination | UE | upper extremity | ~ | approximately |
| Sx | symptom | UMN | upper motor neuron | @ | at |
| T | temperature; Trace (muscle strength grade of 1) | URI | upper respiratory infection | Δ | change |
| | | US | ultrasound | > | greater than |
| T&A | tonsillectomy and adenoidectomy | UTI | urinary tract infection | < | less than |
| | | UV | ultraviolet | = | equals |
| tab | tablet | VC | vital capacity | + | plus; positive (also abbreviated pos.) |
| TAB | therapeutic abortion | VD | venereal disease | | |
| TB | tuberculosis | v.o. | verbal orders | - | minus; negative (also abbreviated neg.) |
| TBI | traumatic brain injury | vol. | volume | | |
| tbsp. | tablespoon | VS | vital signs | # | number (#1); pounds |
| TEDS | thrombo-embolic disease stockings | WBC | white blood cell; white blood count | / | per |
| | | | | % | percent |
| TENS, TNS | transcutaneous electrical nerve stimulator | w/c | wheelchair | +, &, et. | and |
| | | WDWN | well developed, well nourished | ° | degree |
| THR | total hip replacement | | | √ | flexion |
| TIA | transient ischemic attack | wk | week | / | extension |
| | | WFL | within functional limits | ⇆, ↔ | to and from |
| t.i.d. | three times a day | WNL | within normal limits | → | to; progressing forward; approaching |
| TKR | total knee replacement | wt | weight | | |
| TM(J) | temporomandibular (joint) | x1, x2 | assistance (assistance of 1 person given; also written "assistance of 1") Example: "transferred to toilet c̄ min Ⓐ x2" | 1° | primary |
| TNR | tonic neck reflex (also ATNR; STNR) | | | 2° | secondary; secondary to |
| t.o. | telephone order | | | | |
| TPR | temperature, pulse, and respiration | | | | |
| | | y.o. | year old | | |
| TRS | therapeutic recreation specialist | yd. | yard | | |
| | | yr | year | | |
| tsp. | teaspoon | ♂ | male | | |

# WORKSHEET 2-1
## Using Abbreviations

**Translate each sentence written with abbreviations into full English phrases or sentences.**

Pt. c/o pain in Ⓡ MCP joint p̄ ~ 15 min PROM.

Pt. w/c → mat c̄ sliding board max Ⓐ x2.

Pt. Ox4.

Pt. able to don pants SBA c̄ verbal cues to thread Ⓛ LE.

1° dx. THR 2° dx. COPD & CHF.

***Shorten these notes using only the standard abbreviations in your syllabus.***

Patient has thirty degrees of passive range of motion in the left distal interphalangeal joint which is within functional limits.

Patient is able to put on her socks with standby assistance, but requires moderate assistance with putting on and taking off left shoe.

The patient requires contact guard assistance for balance during her morning dressing which she performs while sitting on the edge of her bed.

From Borcherding S. *Documentation Manual for Writing SOAP Notes in Occupational Therapy.* © 2000 SLACK Incorporated

# WORKSHEET 2-2
## Additional Practice

*Shorten these notes using only the standard abbreviations in your syllabus.*

The patient was seen bedside for training in activities of daily living. She was able to perform bed mobility exercises with moderate assistance, but needed maximum assistance to put on her Depends. She was able to go from a supine position to a sitting position with minimum assistance and from a sitting position to a standing position with moderate assistance.

The resident came to the occupational therapy clinic via wheelchair escort. The resident was observed to lean to his left. The resident needed verbal cues and minimum assistance in positioning his body in the wheelchair to maintain midline orientation and symmetrical posture. The resident transferred from his wheelchair to the toilet with moderate assistance of one person using a standing pivot transfer. He needed verbal cues and visual feedback from a mirror to maintain upright posture.

The veteran was seen in his own room seated in a wheelchair for an initial evaluation. The veteran's short-term memory was three out of three for immediate recall, one out of three after one minute, and zero out of three with verbal cues after five minutes. The left upper extremity shoulder flexion was a grade of four, shoulder extension was a grade of four, elbow flexion was a grade of four, elbow extension was a grade of four, wrist extension was a grade of four minus, wrist flexion was a grade of four minus, and grip strength was a eight pounds. The left upper extremity muscle grades are within functional limits and the right upper extremity light touch is intact.

From Borcherding S. *Documentation Manual for Writing SOAP Notes in Occupational Therapy.* © 2000 SLACK Incorporated

# CHAPTER 3
## Writing Functional Problem Statements

After assessing the patient, the occupational therapist develops a "problem list" identifying the major areas that were not within functional limits. Priorities are then set with the patient and family so that the problems that are most important to them will be addressed.

The diagnosis is not the **problem**. For example, if the patient has sustained a head injury, the problem is *not* TBI, but rather the occupational performance areas that are no longer WFL such as:

> *Pt. is unable to carry out ADL tasks due to < 45 second attention span 2° TBI.*

> *Pt. needs mod Ⓐ in dressing due to poor trunk stability.*

In occupational therapy treatment, problems must have a functional component. For ease of writing, you can use the following to write a problem statement:

Pt. _____ in _____ due to _____.
  *Assist level*          *Performing what activity*          *Performance component*

Rather than saying that the patient is unable to perform a given activity, such as bathe lower body independently, it is better to give the assist level needed. In that way, you are able to measure progress as the patient progresses. In other words, if your problem statement reads:

> *Client is unable to dress self Ⓘ due to ↓ AROM in Ⓑ UE.*

An increase in function will not be shown until the patient is independent in dressing. If you word your problem statement to show the amount that the AROM is decreased and the current level of assistance needed:

> *Client needs max Ⓐ in dressing self due to ½ AROM in Ⓑ UE.*

As soon as the patient is able to regain enough active range to dress with mod Ⓐ, or shows an increase in AROM, you can document progress. It may be useful to add the cause, such as:

> *Client needs max Ⓐ in dressing due to ½ AROM in Ⓑ UE 2° to infection of the spinal cord.*

It is not mandatory to add the causative factor. Sometimes it is irrelevant or unknown. It is sometimes helpful since there may be a difference in the treatment that will be provided based on the cause.

Usually if a patient is unable to perform an activity Ⓘ the assist level will be specified. However, sometimes the activity is one that the patient either can or cannot do, with no assist levels in question. In that case, you can use the following format:

Pt. unable to _____ due to _____.
  *Perform what skill*          *Performance component*

For example:
> *Child is unable to do jumping jacks to participate in gym class due to motor planning deficits.*

In this case, the child cannot do the task with any level of assistance. It is a *can or can't* activity. The child is not Ⓓ in jumping jacks, she just can't do them.

It is not mandatory that the above formats be used. These are useful ways of wording, but there are others. Sometimes a slightly different format is more useful:

_____ results in _____.
*Limiting factor*                    *What functional deficit*

For example:

*Decreased Ⓡ UE sensation results in inability to perform self-care activities safely.*

*Pain level > 6 at end ranges limits ability to move through full AROM to participate in self-care.*

> Note: Just as a humanitarian reminder, please write in terms of what the patient needs, rather than stating that the patient is a particular assist level. Our patients *are* much more than a particular assist level. In this manual you will find the patient referred to as "patient, client, consumer, veteran, child, resident or individual" in various notes. All of these are commonly used and vary by facility. Please use the term that is considered most respectful in your setting.

Please say:
    *Veteran needs or requires max assist...*
Rather than:
    *Veteran is max assist...*

Please say:
    *Individual will dress with mod assist...*
Rather than:
    *Individual will be mod assist in dressing...*

The language we use in speaking of patients reminds us that they are more than their disabilities or limitations and deserve our respect.

# Examples of Functional Problem Statements

## Cognition

*Impaired short-term memory makes patient unsafe in home management tasks.*

*Pt. requires mod physical assist with upper body dressing 2° to attention span of < 5 minutes.*

*Individual requires verbal and tactile cues 100% of the time in order to stay on task, initiate, and sequence during dressing activity.*

## Communication

*Veteran unable to communicate verbally 2° intubation.*

## Dressing

*Client requires mod assist to don pants 2° 3+ upper extremity strength.*

*Pt. requires mod Ⓐ with UE dressing 2° Ⓑ UE strength of 2/5.*

*Pt. requires mod verbal cues and mod physical assist with upper body dressing 2° attention span of < 5 minutes.*

## Endurance (Activity Tolerance)

*Patient tolerates <10 minutes ADL activity secondary to shortness of breath.*

*Client unsafe in home management tasks due to inability to recognize fatigue when standing.*

## Feeding

*Individual unable to keep food on fork due to poor motor planning.*

*Resident requires set up for feeding 2° blindness in both eyes.*

*Child unable to feed self due to asymmetrical positioning in wheelchair.*

## Grooming/Self-Care

*Patient requires mod Ⓐ in dressing and hygiene activities 2° legal blindness.*

*Veteran requires max Ⓐ in combing hair with Ⓡ UE due to pain in Ⓡ elbow.*

*Client unsafe and mod Ⓐ in bathing 2° poor balance and lack of adaptive equipment.*

## Hands

*Child needs mod Ⓐ in upper body hygiene 2° pronator spasticity which limits supination of Ⓡ forearm by ½ range.*

*Pt. is unable to do carpentry work due to grip strength of 4# in Ⓡ hand.*

## Mobility/Transfers

*Resident needs max Ⓐ in bed mobility secondary to decreased strength in trunk and UEs.*

*Veteran requires mod Ⓐ in transfers due to trunk instability.*

*Client Ⓓ in bed mobility due to severe UE and LE contractures.*

## Pain

*Pain level of > 6/10 at end ranges limits ability to move through full AROM to participate in self-care.*

*Pt. unable to grasp and hold tool with Ⓛ hand due to pain level > 5/10 with flexion of Ⓛ index finger.*

*Pain level of > 5/10 with flexion of Ⓡ fingers makes patient unable to grasp a writing instrument for more than 3 minutes.*

## Pediatrics

*Patient unable to do jumping jacks during recess as a result of poor motor planning.*

*Pt. requires mod Ⓐ to complete art assignment requiring the use of a ruler 2° bilateral uncoordination.*

## Safety

*Patient has history of falls with continued risk for falls during shower.*

*Impaired short-term memory makes client unsafe to cook or care for young children.*

*Patient unsafe in cooking tasks due to impaired judgment and sequencing.*

## Sensation

*Decreased Ⓡ UE sensation results in mod Ⓐ to perform self-care activities independently or safely.*

## Upper Extremity Use

*Decreased fine motor manipulation in Ⓛ UE causes AM routine to require 1½ hours.*

*<60° AROM in Ⓡ shoulder abduction limits patient's ability to use Ⓡ UE for upper body ADL and work tasks.*

*Client needs adaptive equipment in order to return to carpentry work 2° to ↓ sensation in thumb and index finger 2° to C 5-6 lesion.*

*Trace strength in shoulder, elbow, and wrist flexors/extensors 2°Ⓛ CVA results in need for mod Ⓐ in showering safely.*

## Mental Health

*Consumer's low self-esteem puts her at risk for suicide.*

*Individual's aggressive behavior results in social isolation.*

## Substance Abuse

*Client has been using alcohol and drugs on a regular basis for at least 1 year, resulting in inability to complete home management tasks.*

*Consumer admits to using cocaine on a daily basis resulting in inability to hold a job.*

## Problem Statements in Mental Health and Substance Abuse

Although goals for mental health and substance abuse can be written in this format, as shown above, in practice they are often done as a two-part statement. For example:

*Problem:*                                         Alcohol use
*Behavioral Manifestations:*       *Bill admits to drinking 8 oz. of liquor and seven to eight beers nightly, resulting in failing grades and involvement with the law due to fighting with fists and weapons.*

For more examples of problem statements in mental health and chemical dependency, see Chapter 11.

# WORKSHEET 3-1

## Writing Functional Problem Statements

Please use the following problems to write functional problem statements. Make them specific enough to:
- Show both the performance areas and the performance components which are not WFL
- Serve as a baseline against which to measure progress

1.    The client has acquired an injury to his brain. As a result, he is not able to pay attention to tasks for very long period of time, and is having trouble completing his morning routine. Usually he can pay attention to what he is doing for about 2 minutes, and needs to be redirected back to the task after that.

2.    The resident is not very cognitively aware. She has trouble figuring out what to do first if she has to complete a complex task, and she doesn't remember what she has just been told.

3.    Mr. J. has recently sustained a Ⓡ CVA. His Ⓛ upper extremity is flaccid and he forgets it is there.

4.    The patient is unable to transfer w/c ⇆ toilet by himself. One of the primary reasons he can't transfer is because he must observe total hip precautions. In addition, there are strength and balance problems.

5.    The veteran has increased tone in his formerly dominant Ⓡ upper extremity. He is referred to OT to work on ADL tasks.

# CHAPTER 4
## Writing Functional and Measurable Goals and Objectives

Goals and objectives used in a treatment plan must be written in functional, measurable, observable, action-oriented terms. They must also be realistic for the patient, and able to be achieved in a "reasonable" amount of time. Goals are formulated from the problem list you have compiled, in collaboration with the patient. For successful treatment, it is critical that you work on goals that are important to the patient. Occupational therapy goals must focus on functional gains. The component or biomechanical gains that underlie such progress are much less important to a third party payer than what the patient can actually do, even though the gains in performance components may be essential to achieving the functional outcome.

**Goals** in a treatment plan are also called "long-term goals" (LTG) or outcomes. These are usually discharge goals—what the therapist hopes to see the patient accomplish by the time of discharge. For each problem you have identified, you will have at least one long-term goal, and often more than one.

**Objectives** are also called "short-term goals" (STG). These are the daily goals that are met while progressing toward the discharge goals.

For example, if your LTG is:

> *In order to perform a job without injury, pt. will be able to move 35# objects needed for work from table to counter without ↑ in pain by 12/18/99.*

Then one of your STGs might be:

> *In order to perform tasks of job, pt. will be able to lift 10# objects needed for work without increase in pain by 12/5/99.*

If your LTG is:

> *In order to return to independent living situation, pt. will transfer independently and safely bed ⇆ wheelchair standing pivot, and wearing an orthotic foot support within 2 weeks.*

Then one of your STGs might be:

> *In order to be independent and safe in standing pivot transfers required for returning home, pt. will reach for bed or wheelchair before sitting with no verbal cues within 1 week.*

You may have several STGs (objectives) for each LTG. For example, suppose you are treating Mr. Hawkins, a 45-year-old executive who sustained a Ⓡ CVA a few days ago and has Ⓛ side hemiplegia. On evaluation you find that he is oriented X 4, verbal, intelligent, able to learn, and has a supportive wife. After talking with him about what he would like to achieve in OT, you and he decide upon a goal of independent upper body dressing. You believe that this is a realistic goal, provided he receives skilled instruction and the correct adaptive equipment.

You set a series of objectives:
1. In order to begin dressing activities, patient will be able to maintain dynamic sitting balance at edge of bed for > 5 minutes while reaching for clothing at arm's length by the end of the 3rd treatment session.
2. By the 6th treatment session, patient will be able to tolerate >10 minutes of dressing sitting edge of bed.
3. After skilled instruction, patient will be able to don shirt sitting EOB using the over the head method by 3/10/99.

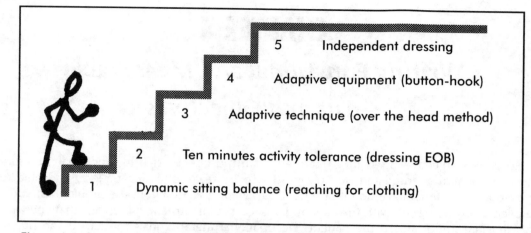

5    Independent dressing

4    Adaptive equipment (button-hook)

3    Adaptive technique (over the head method)

2    Ten minutes activity tolerance (dressing EOB)

1    Dynamic sitting balance (reaching for clothing)

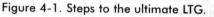

Figure 4-1. Steps to the ultimate LTG.

4.      After skilled instruction, patient will be able to button shirt using a button-hook by 3/12/99.

5.      While sitting on edge of bed, patient will be independent in upper body dressing by 3/15/99.

As you can see, each of these STGs is measurable, observable, and client-action oriented. The first four STGs are steps to the ultimate LTG.

A treatment plan is always a work in progress. There are events and conditions that you may not expect that can impact the progress your patient will be able to make toward his or her goals. If you find a goal unrealistic, you are obligated to change. It is not useful to continue with a plan that is not working.

For example, suppose that your patient, Mr. Hawkins, begins to have some return in his involved Ⓛ upper extremity. You now know that he may be able to dress his upper body without adaptive techniques or equipment, and he wants very much to do that. After we discuss the format for writing goals, you might write a new set of short-term goals for Mr. Hawkins.

In order to write goals and objectives in a way that can be measured, the elements to be included are very specific. The FEAST method is useful as you are learning to write (Table 4-1). The order may need to be changed slightly in order for your sentence to make sense. As long as all the required elements are present, you can begin with any of the elements—the expectation, the conditions, the timeline, or the function. Now let's look at each category a little more closely.

# F (Function)

This is the specific performance area to which this goal pertains, if it is not imbedded in the goal. For example: "...in order to be able to dress self with minimum assist," or "in order to return to work as a carpenter," or "in order to be able to be bathed by his caretakers," or "in order to be able to write his name."

For example:

*In order to begin writing his name, the student will demonstrate ability to hold a crayon using tripod pinch by 3/19/99.*

The function may go after the action if you prefer. For example:

*The student will be able to hold a crayon using tripod pinch in order to learn to write his name by 3/19/99.*

Often the function is the same as the action.

*The patient will perform a three step cooking process at wheelchair level by 3/16/99.*

In this case the function (cooking) is inherent in the goal and does not need to be restated.

Function is the core of occupational therapy practice. It is the **first** thing you think of in writing goals, and should be the essential focus of the goal statement.

```
┌─────────────────────────────────────────────────────────────┐
│                                                               │
│                        Table 4-1                              │
│                Goal Writing: FEAST Method                     │
│                                                               │
│        F—Function            For what functional gain?        │
│        E—Expectation         The patient will?                │
│        A—Action              Do what?                         │
│        S—Specific Conditions Under what conditions?           │
│        T—Timeline            By when?                         │
│                                                               │
└─────────────────────────────────────────────────────────────┘
```

# E (Expectation)

In writing treatment goals, the patient is the key player. You set the expectation:

*The patient will...*

# A (Action)

Note: These are the patient's goals. The goal statement is **not** the place to tell what the therapist will do. That goes later, under intervention strategies.

An action verb is inserted here such as perform, demonstrate, identify, cook, don, comb, unfasten or complete, followed by the skill to be performed. For example:

*The patient will perform a three step cooking process.*

Usually the function is contained in the action statement, and does not need to be added.

# S (Specific Conditions)

This is the level of assistance expected and/or the conditions under which the patient is expected to be able to perform the desired action. For example: "...after set up"; "...by using a dressing stick"; "...at wheelchair level"; "...after skilled instruction."

*The patient will perform a three step cooking process at wheelchair level...*

The conditions make your goal more specific. Usually it is helpful to put the condition after the skill rather than before it, but sometimes you may want to start with the condition. For example:

*After skilled instruction the patient will be able to perform a three step cooking process...*

The following are some examples of goals in which the conditions have been highlighted for emphasis. One of the most common mistakes in goal writing is omission of the conditions under which the activity is expected to be performed.

*In order to dress himself with minimum assistance, pt. will button at least three buttons on his shirt using a button-hook by 3/1/96.*

*In order to be able to begin dressing training by 11/30/97, pt. will maintain static sitting balance ① for 3 minutes on side of bed.*

*After skilled instruction, pt. will demonstrate proper use of sock-aid to don socks Ⓘ safely while seated in w/c by end of 6th treatment session.*

*In order to don pants completely over hips pt. will demonstrate ability to transfer sit ⇆ stand Ⓘ within 4 weeks.*

# T (Timeline)

This is the time frame within which the goal is expected to be accomplished. For example: "...by discharge on 3/16/99" or "...by the end of the next treatment session," or "...within 2 weeks."

*The patient will perform a three step cooking process at wheelchair level by 3/16/99.*

# Medical Necessity

As occupational therapists we are trained to view a patient holistically, considering the "whole person" with his needs, interests, problems, strengths, and priorities rather than focusing in on a "faulty part" of the mechanism. We know that leisure is an important part of the total picture. When this is the patient's priority, we might be inclined to write goals focusing on leisure skills and interests. For example:

**Problem:**    *Pt. unable to play softball due to ↓ AROM and ↑ pain in Ⓛ wrist.*
**LTG:**    *In order to resume his role as a team member of a softball team, pt. will demonstrate AROM of the Ⓛ wrist WFL without pain within 6 weeks.*
**STG:**    *In order to prepare for resuming his role as a softball team member, pt. will demonstrate wrist stabilization for 1 minute while holding a 1# ball within 2 weeks.*

As knowledgeable health care professionals, we also know that both Medicare and managed care organizations are very frugal with our health care dollars and approve expenditures only for medical necessity. Since even adaptive equipment such as a raised toilet seat is not always considered medically necessary, treatment focused on the patient's leisure goals is likely to be denied under our current reimbursement system. In consideration of the patient's total needs and the reimbursement considerations, we may address in the treatment plan performance components that enable the patient to perform a variety of functional tasks. Documentation would include treatment that provides the patient with skills for self-care and work activities and also leisure activities so important to the quality of life.

In the example above, we might suspect that the patient is having difficulty with household or work tasks requiring Ⓑ upper body use as well as having trouble playing ball. It would work much better to choose IADL tasks which also require ↑ AROM and the ability to hold a 1# object for 1 minute as goals, knowing that improving these performance components would also give the patient an increased ability to pursue his leisure interests.

# WORKSHEET 4-1

## *Choosing Goals for Medical Necessity*

**Problem:**    Pt. unable to perform sewing due to 2+ strength in Ⓡ hand musculature.
**LTG:**         Pt. will be able to perform embroidery Ⓘ for 20 minutes within 5 months.
**STG:**         In order to ↑ performance of embroidery, pt. will be able to use needle continuously for 5 minutes  by 11/6/98.

**What other problems might this woman have due to decreased strength in her Ⓡ hand?**

**What LTG might you use that would show medical necessity for increasing  Ⓡ  UE strength?**

**What short-term goal might be used as a step to that LTG?**

Stringent requirements necessitate documentation that demonstrates a clear indication of the need for skilled occupational therapy. Activities that require only minimal assistance may lead to denial of payment unless the necessity of skilled occupational therapy is specified. For example, dressing with minimal assist does not necessarily indicate a need for skilled occupational therapy. However "minimal assistance with verbal instruction for over-the-head method of donning of shirt" justifies skilled occupational therapy.

## Educational Goals

Therapists working in the public schools use a slightly different terminology. In education, goals for one school year are called "objectives." Educational goals are not measured by time, that is, by 5/7/99 or within 3 weeks. Since the IEP is rewritten annually, the time frame for educational goals is assumed to be annual. Children sometimes exhibit a new behavior inconsistently before it is really established. Therefore, measurement used for children is more likely to reflect whether or not the behavior is established. For example:

*Kevin will hold pencil in a tripod grasp in 3/3 opportunities.*

*Johnny will demonstrate improved tolerance to tactile media as evidenced by self-initiation during art activities in 5/5 teacher reports.*

Goals for children in the public schools must be set in terms of a behavior that is needed in the classroom. While you may be working on sensory integration as a treatment goal such as maintaining prone extension posture over a therapy ball, it must be written in language that relates to performance in the classroom setting.

*Bobby will maintain upright sitting posture during writing time without verbal reminders in 3/3 observations.*

**Do not** use participation in treatment as a goal. For example:

*Pt. will do 20 reps of shoulder ladder with 1# wt. in order to ↑ endurance to become more Ⓘ in ADLs.*

In a goal such as this, specify the amount of ↑ endurance you hope or expect to see. For example:

*Pt. will be able to participate in cooking task >5 minutes without rest breaks.*

# Examples of Well-Written Goal Statements

## ADL Skills

*Pt. will be able to unfasten 3 out of 4 buttons Ⓘ within 2 weeks.*

*Pt. will don socks with CGA using a sock-aid by 9/8/98.*

## Cognition

*Pt. will feed self a meal with correct use of adaptive equipment (lipped plate, rocker knife, and built-up angled utensils) after set up with no more than 10 verbal cues by 9-11-99.*

*Pt. will perform grooming with less than 3 verbal cues to redirect attention to task within 1 week.*

*In order to grocery shop Ⓘ, pt. will locate proper aisle within 5 minutes of entering grocery store.*

## Edema

*Pt. will independently implement edema control techniques during work routine by 4/9/99.*

*In order to return to work as a typist, pt. will demonstrate 10% reduction in wrist circumference within 3 treatment sessions.*

## Activity Tolerance

*In order to complete morning ADL tasks pt. will tolerate >10 minutes of activity with no more than one rest period by 10/19/99.*

*In order to perform grooming tasks Ⓘ, pt. will tolerate >5 minutes of activity with Ⓛ hand with a reported pain level of less than 3/10 within 3 tx. sessions.*

## Pain

*Pt. will comb hair Ⓘ s̄ c/o pain by the 5th treatment session.*

*Pt. will complete grooming and hygiene activities with a reported pain level of >3/10 within 3 tx. sessions.*

## Range of Motion

Biomechanical goals are no longer used in many areas of clinical practice because of payment issues. Use functional goals instead, if possible.

*Pt. will demonstrate ↑ shoulder flexion PROM to 90° and abduction to 50° in order to don shirt with min Ⓐ in 2 weeks.*

*In order to perform button shirt Ⓘ , pt. will demonstrate Ⓡ thumb MP flexion of no less than 50° within 2 weeks.*

## Return to Work

*In order to return to carpentry work, pt. will demonstrate Ⓡ UE grip strength >70# within 4 weeks.*

## Safety

*After skilled instruction, patient will demonstrate an ability to shower safely using adaptive equipment with mod Ⓐ within 2 weeks.*

*In order to return to living unassisted, patient will demonstrate an ability to locate phone numbers of emergency services in the telephone directory without physical or verbal cues after the 3rd treatment session.*

## Transfers/Mobility

*Within 4 weeks, pt. will perform a pivot transfer mod Ⓐ from bed to wheelchair in order to be Ⓘ in toileting.*

*In order to return to living at home, pt. will be able to propel w/c up ramp and through all doors with min. Ⓐ within 2 weeks.*

## Mental Health and Substance Abuse

*Consumer will Ⓘ prepare a TV dinner in the microwave within 1 week.*

*Consumer will Ⓘ request a job application from a restaurant within 1 week.*

*Consumer will take a shower without prompting at least 4x wk. by 7/12/99.*

*With mod verbal cues, consumer will ask roommate to smoke outside the building.*

*Client will develop a plan for leisure time that does not include drinking by 4/8/99.*

# WORKSHEET 4-2

## Evaluating Goal Statements

Which of the following goals has each of the necessary components to be useful in occupational therapy documentation?  For each goal that you find to be incomplete or inaccurate in some way, indicate what it lacks.

1.      By the time of discharge in 2 weeks, patient will be able to dress himself with min
        Ⓐ for balance using a sock aid and reacher while sitting in a wheelchair.
        __ This goal has all the necessary components to be useful
        __ This goal lacks _____

2.      Patient will tolerate 10 minutes of treatment daily.
        __ This goal has all the necessary components to be useful
        __ This goal lacks _____

3.      Patient will demonstrate increased coping skills in order to live at home with her
        granddaughter within 2 weeks.
        __ This goal has all the necessary components to be useful
        __ This goal lacks _____

4.      Patient will demonstrate 15 minutes of activity tolerance without rest breaks
        using Ⓑ UE in order to complete ADL tasks before breakfast each morning.
        __ This goal has all the necessary components to be useful
        __ This goal lacks _____

5.      In order to be able to toilet self Ⓘ after discharge, patient will demonstrate abili-
        ty to perform a sliding board transfer w/c ⇆ mat within the next week.
        __ This goal has all the necessary components to be useful
        __ This goal lacks _____

6.      OT will teach lower body dressing using a reacher, dressing stick, and sock aid
        within 3 tx. sessions.
        __ This goal has all the necessary components to be useful
        __ This goal lacks _____

7.      In order to return to living independently, pt. will demonstrate ability to balance
        his checkbook.
        __ This goal has all the necessary components to be useful
        __ This goal lacks _____

# WORKSHEET 4-3

## Writing Realistic, Functional Measurable Goals

Rewrite the following goals to be measurable, functional, time limited, and action oriented, and specifying the conditions under which the action is to occur. Without knowing more details about the patient, it is impossible to know what the goal would be. For purposes of this exercise, just imagine a patient and decide what the goal might be, then practice wording it correctly.

1.      **Increase attention span**
        F (if not included in action below)_____
        *(For what functional gain)*

        E _____
        *(Expectation—the patient will)*

        A _____
        *(Action)*

        S _____
        *(Specific Conditions)*

        T _____
        *(Time line—by when?)*

2.      **Teach the patient to follow directions**
        F (if not included in action below)_____

        E _____

        A _____

        S _____

        T _____

3.      **Pt. to dress upper body**
        F (if not included in action below)_____

        E _____

        A _____

        S _____

        T _____

4.      **Increase endurance**
        F (if not included in action below)_____

        E _____

        A _____

        S _____

        T _____

5.      **Improve money management skills**
        F (if not included in action below)_____

        E _____

        A _____

        S _____

        T _____

6.      **Decrease depression**
        F (if not included in action below)_____

        E _____

        A _____

        S _____

        T _____

# CHAPTER 5
## Writing the "S"—Subjective

There are many correct ways to write notes using the SOAP format. In this manual, you will be learning a formula that works. It is not the only correct method. You may find that your supervising therapist does it quite differently and the therapist's method may be very useful. You will eventually develop your own style of writing. However, for purposes of this manual we will do notes using the SOAP formula.

## S (Subjective)

The first section is **Subjective**. In this section the therapist records the patient's report of limitations, concerns, and problems. Subjective data is information that cannot be verified or measured during the evaluation. In this section, you document what the patient said that was relevant to treatment, such as significant complaints like pain, fatigue, or expressions of feelings, attitudes, concerns, goals, and plans. You may use a quote or summarize what the patient said.

For example:

*Pt. communicated using her message board that she wanted to be able to take care of herself.*

*Resident reports pain in ® shoulder.*

*Patient asked for help when it was needed during dressing.*

*Patient reports, "I can't wash the dishes or zip my coat."*

*Veteran reports that his fingers "look kind of dead."*

*Consumer says, "I don't need therapy."*

*Pt. reported he needed to go to meet someone and get to work when the session began. When asked questions such as "can you hear me?" he often responded, "I need to go."*

*Resident reports he feels "pretty good" now and his goal is to "get back as natural" as he can.*

*Pt. reports that his doctor has ordered some home care for "a few days to work on transfers."*

*During the initial OT session, client reported, "I keep blowing up at home, and yelling at everyone, and I don't know what to do about it."*

*Client answered questions and reported that her shoulders feel better after taping. "My short-term goal is to return to work, and my long-term goal is to be able to write," she said.*

*Pt. described her previous medical history, including the fall that fractured her ® ankle. She reports living with her daughter and having an attendant stay with her when her daughter is at work. Pt. reports having a hospital bed as well as a trapeze, walker, and 3-in-1 commode. She reports having four steps leading into her home, with hand rails on both sides.*

*Client reports being able to bathe and dress self Ⓘ , but does not open dresser drawers and closet doors due to a fall from opening a dresser drawer which resulted in a hip fracture. She was able to tell the correct day and month when asked.*

*Patient commented that she used her Ⓛ hand to hold a cup but now is unable to do so. Pt. also inquired about finding a student to assist her at home upon discharge. Client also complained of soreness in Ⓛ shoulder and stated that she has experienced several episodes of bladder incontinence when trying to make it to the bathroom.*

*Martha called the emergency line last night to report a burning sensation in her "gut" which made her afraid she was going to die. Today she reports that she has been worrying about dying and has not showered since the day before yesterday.*

*Consumer contributed to ~ 98% of the group discussion, reporting that the hardest feelings for her to deal with are worry and fear about her physical problems, which might go undetected. She reports being unable to function at home (cannot cook, keep house, or do laundry) when she is sick with depression, but wants to do these things again. Consumer reports that exercise, prayer, and volunteer work are her primary coping strategies, and that she would like to learn more about relaxation techniques.*

Sometimes the patient is not able to speak or does not make any relevant comments. In such cases include that information in the "S" section.

For example:

*Patient unable to communicate due to aphasia.*

*Patient did not speak without cuing.*

*Resident does not clearly verbalize during treatment, but smiles and nods appropriately when asked questions.*

Occasionally you will include information that the nursing staff or family said about the patient, however, the "S" section is usually reserved for the patient's view.

# Common Errors

The most common error that new therapists make is in failing to use interviewing skills effectively during the treatment session, instead using the time to talk socially. A good interview is at the heart of your assessment and establishes a relationship that allows you to provide effective treatment. Instead of talking to your patient about the weather or Monday Night Football, why not talk about how he feels treatment is going or the psychosocial issues he faces at discharge? As therapists gain experience, they begin to use the treatment session to further evaluate the patient by skillful interviewing and assessing such things as functional status, prior level of functioning, motivation, priorities, and family support.

A well-done interview seems just like a conversation on the surface. You as a skilled therapist direct the conversation to topics that are meaningful to patient care rather than allowing it to remain superficial. Use this opportunity to update and gather data that is vital to providing the very best occupational therapy possible. In having a conversation with your patient, guide the discussion to your patient's history, problems, needs, strengths, support systems, living situation, and goals for treatment. Without knowing these things from your patient's point of view, you will have difficulty planning effective treatment. When a therapist does not listen effectively during treatment, the "S" may read:

> *Patient talked about grandchildren visiting.*
> **- OR -**
> *Pt. said "ouch" when elbow was ranged beyond 45°.*

While these statements are within the scope of the "S," they are not particularly helpful pieces of information to spend time and space reporting.

## Being More Coherent

The second most common error made by new therapists in writing the subjective section of the note is that of simply listing anything important the patient had to say about his condition.

For example:

> *Pt. remarked, "I can't feel anything with my hands."*

> *Pt. stated, "I'm wobbly as all get out today."*

> *Pt. expressed dizziness after bending down to touch the floor while in a seated position. Pt. acknowledged improvement in his sitting balance in comparison to the previous week.*

Many of these statements have to do with stability, balance, and safety. While the quotations are a very objective way of reporting the data and all the statements are relative to the treatment session, the same data could have been reported in a more concise and coherent manner.

---

Write a more concise and organized version of this "S".

# WORKSHEET 5-1
## Choosing a Subjective Statement

The following observation was made by an occupational therapy student treating a patient.

*Pt. seen in rehab clinic for UE activities to ↑ AROM in Ⓡ shoulder, activity tolerance, UE strength, and dynamic standing balance, in order to ↑ independence in ADL tasks.*

*ADL: Pt. seen in room for instruction in safety techniques and adaptive equipment use in toileting. Pt. needs bilateral grab bars in bathroom to sit ⇆ stand safely. Pt. attempted to stand while pulling on walker and one grab bar. Pt. was instructed on safety issues and the use of bilateral grab bars.*

*Performance Components: Pt. sit → stand CGA for balance. Pt. worked on activity tolerance, dynamic standing balance, and ↑ AROM in Ⓡ shoulder by moving canned goods from counter to cupboard for 5 minutes before needing a 2 minute sitting rest. After resting, she poured liquid from a pitcher while standing CGA for balance. After 1 minute rest, pt. pushed wheeled walker while picking up objects from the floor with a reacher in order to increase dynamic standing balance and safety in ADL activities. AROM in right shoulder abduction < 90°. PROM right shoulder abduction WNL.*

**The treatment session included all of the following. Which would be best to use as the subjective section of your note?**

1.   Patient was cooperative and engaged in social conversation throughout the treatment session.

2.   Patient remarked that her grandson will be coming to visit later in the week, and that she will be very glad to see him.

3.   Patient reports that she feels "pretty good" today.

4.   Patient says she is unable to move right UE, although she does not know why it will not move. She reports, "It really doesn't hurt. It's just tight."

5.   Nursing staff report patient is unsafe to toilet self independently.

# CHAPTER 6
## Writing the "O"—Objective

The second section of the note is **Objective** where you will record all measurable, quantifiable, and observable data obtained during the treatment session. In this section you will present a picture of the treatment session you have observed.

## Organization of the "O"

There are different ways that are acceptable in organizing this information. You may choose to present the information chronologically, discussing each treatment event in the order it occurred during that treatment session.

> O:     Pt. seen in clinic for wheelchair positioning. Foot guard attached to prevent Ⓛ foot from dropping behind/between footrests. New wedge cushion c̄ dycem inserted on both sides to prevent slipping. Wedge pillow placed on Ⓛ side for lateral support. Longer safety restraint placed around pt.'s trunk, replacing tighter one. Folded blanket placed between pt.'s knees. Family via a phone call and staff educated on pt.'s positioning changes and goals.

Alternately, you may choose to organize your information into categories.

> O:     Pt. seen in clinic kitchen for skilled instruction in a cooking task.
>
> **Mobility:** Pt. maneuvered throughout kitchen in w/c with verbal cues to place w/c in appropriate position for reaching objects in kitchen. Pt. min. Ⓐ in stabilizing items while transporting items in lap and maneuvering w/c simultaneously.
>
> **UE ROM and strength:** WFL for reaching items in drawers, opening oven door, and putting dishes in the sink Ⓘ. UE strength adequate for opening refrigerator door and stirring batter Ⓘ. Pt. requires min. Ⓐ in opening plastic container.
>
> **Hand function and strength:** Adequate for unscrewing lids, cracking egg, and opening muffin box. Pt. able to use necessary tools for carrying out task Ⓘ. Pt. able to set oven dial and put muffins in oven Ⓘ.
>
> **Activity tolerance:** Pt. took 3-minute break after ~ 20 minutes of activity Ⓘ.
>
> **Cognition:** Pt. able to respond to verbal instructions and questions with correct response 3/3 times. Pt. said she did not think it would be safe for her to take the muffins out of the oven. Pt. able to problem-solve Ⓘ about repositioning her w/c 75% of tx. time.

When categorizing your information, choose the categories that make sense for your note. There is no list of "correct" categories. Whether you choose to report the treatment session chronologically or divide your information into sections, you may want to consider noting some of the following:

- **Specifics of ADL Performance**
  Setting of the session, type of clothing, shaver, etc. Include Assist levels including set up, any adaptive equipment or technique used, UE or LE. Also include type of cuing and response, training/assessment positioning, special equipment, and how the various performance components affect function.

- **The Patient's Posture and Balance**
  Does the patient lean in one direction? Is his posture rotated? How is the weight distributed? What is the position of the head? Facial expression? Symmetry?

- **The Patient's Coordination**
  Hand dominance, type of prehension used, ability to grasp and maintain grasp without dropping, gross vs. fine motor ability.

- **Swelling or Edema**
  Give girth or volumetric measurements if possible, pitting or non-pitting including levels if pitting.

- **Movement Patterns Observed in Affected Upper Extremity**
  Tone, tremors, synergy pattern, facilitation required, stabilization, body movement.

- **Ability to Follow Instructions**
  Type and amount of instruction required, such as physical, verbal, or visual cuing, ability to follow one, and two or three step directions.

- **The Patient's Cognitive Status**
  Initiation of task, verbal responses, approach to the task, ability to stay on task, sequencing, oriented x 4, requirements for cuing, number of steps successfully completed in task, judgment (recognition of impairments, impulsivity), ability to respond to written or verbal directions.

- **Neurological Factors**
  Perseveration (motor, speech), sensory losses (specific), motor deficit, praxis, damage to innervation (spasticity, flaccidity, rigidity, synergy), unilateral neglect, bilateral integration, tremors.

- **Performance Components**
  ROM (active, passive, assistive) and why limited, strength (grade and extremity), endurance (time, repetition, signs of fatigue, sitting/standing), coordination (one or two handed, grip, grasp and release, object manipulation), sensation.

- **The Patient's Mobility Status**
  What kind of assistance is needed for the patient to walk or propel his wheelchair (equipment, adapted technique, stand-by, verbal cues) (O'Hara, 1990).

## Observations in Different Practice Settings

In a **mental health** setting, of course, you will be observing psychosocial factors as well as functional ability.

> Client attended anger management group today with verbal prompting by nursing staff and security aides. He displayed his displeasure at being asked to attend the group by using profanity. During the group, client related two instances in which individuals on the unit consistently bother him, and discussed the way he usually handles this situation. Peer feedback was given on other possible ways he might handle the same situation.

In a **pediatric** setting, the child's play or school activities are a part of her activities of daily living.

> Mary was seen in her home to work on ⑬ tasks to ↑ spontaneous use of ⓛ hand as a functional assist, as well as sitting balance as prerequisites to ① in self-care and play skills.
>
> Bilateral UE use: Mary required mod. Ⓐ to pull shirt over stuffed animal's arm. She spontaneously used ⓛ hand to pull/stabilize animal while pulling shirt over its arm and shoulder with ⓡ hand. She initiated snapping shirt, and used ⑬ UEs to hold shirt, but required max Ⓐ to fasten snaps. Mary used both hands to hold animal during play.
>
> Sitting balance: Mary requires touch cues stand → sit in walker, and mod. physical Ⓐ sit → cross leg sit. She demonstrated adequate sitting balance to play for 5 minutes, but after 5 minutes needed two tactile cues to sit up from forward leaning position.

In the **school system**, all activities must be related to school functioning.

> *Student was seen in classroom to work on letter recognition and formation. After proprioceptive input, she was able to identify and match upper and lower case letters with 90% accuracy and min. verbal cues to verbalize answers. She required mod. verbal cues and demonstration to form lower case letters correctly.*

## The Specifics of Writing the "O"

First, begin with a statement about the setting and purpose of the activity.

Pt. seen_____ for _____.
              *In what setting*                            *Purpose of the treatment session*

If the session is centered on working on performance components such as strengthening, range of motion, activity tolerance, or dynamic balance, then add a functional component to the opening sentence.

Pt. seen _____ for _____, _____.
        *Setting*          *Purpose*            *For what expected functional gain*

For example:

> *Resident seen bedside for ADL evaluation.*

> *Client seen in room to provide skilled instruction in energy conservation and for explanation of patient education materials on energy conservation.*

> *Patient seen in outpatient clinic to increase functional movements and prehension patterns of Ⓛ hand in order to prepare for return to work.*

> *Child seen in therapy room to ↑ strength and tone needed to improve handwriting.*

Next, follow the opening sentence of the "O" with either a chronologic rendition of the session, or a categorized summary, focusing on the patient's response to the treatment provided, rather than on what the therapist did. For example:

| | |
|---|---|
| ***Rather than saying:*** | *Patient was reminded about hip precautions.* |
| ***You might say:*** | *Attempting to don shoes, pt. required repeated instruction to keep hip in correct alignment.* |
| ***Rather than saying:*** | *Patient was asked orientation questions pertaining to the time of day.* |
| ***You might say:*** | *When verbally cued to look at watch, patient was unable to correctly identify time.* |
| ***Rather than saying:*** | *Patient demonstrated a postural drift backward and to the left several times while sitting on the edge of the mat.* |
| ***You might say:*** | *Patient required verbal and tactile cues to correct postural drift backward and to the left 4 times in 5 minutes while sitting edge of mat.* |

Always write from the patient's point of view, leaving yourself out. For example:

| | |
|---|---|
| *Rather than saying:* | The occupational therapist put the patient's shoes on for him. |
| *You might say:* | Pt. Ⓓ in donning shoes. |

| | |
|---|---|
| *Rather than saying:* | OT instructed the client and family in energy conservation techniques. |
| *You might say:* | Client and family instructed in energy conservation techniques and demonstrated understanding by performing correctly. |

Make certain that it is clear that you were not just a passive observer in the session.

| | |
|---|---|
| *Rather than saying:* | Client compensated for shoulder flexion by leaning forward with whole body during prehension activities. |
| *You might say:* | Client required skilled instruction to avoid compensation at the shoulder during prehension activities. |

| | |
|---|---|
| *Rather than saying:* | Patient performed Home Exercise Program. |
| *You might say:* | Home Exercise Program was observed for accurate movement patterns and updated to accommodate for progress. |

Although you will assess the information you observed and make a professional judgment about it, avoid judging the patient.

| | |
|---|---|
| *Rather than saying:* | Patient was compliant. **or** Patient was cooperative. |
| *You might say:* | Patient demonstrated ability to follow 3-step directions and sequence WFL. |

Be professional and concise in your wording.

| | |
|---|---|
| *Rather than saying:* | Veteran used a trapeze to sit up. |
| *You might say:* | Supine → sit using trapeze. |

| | |
|---|---|
| *Rather than saying:* | Client placed the board to make a sliding board transfer. |
| *You might say:* | Client positioned sliding board for transfer. |

| | |
|---|---|
| *Rather than saying:* | Resident flopped down onto bed short of breath, closed her eyes, and moaned. Resident laid in bed with min. Ⓐ to position herself. |
| *You might say:* | Pt. observed to be fatigued following tx. session and required min. Ⓐ for positioning in bed. |

## Focus on Function

**Make certain that function is integral to the note.** In a treatment session devoted to ADL evaluation or training, function is obvious. However, in a session devoted to treating performance components such as strength, range and endurance or in a session where modalities are used or in a co-treatment session, **function must be addressed** separately in order to justify skilled occupational therapy. For example, although the note below is an observation of a session that was devoted to performance components, it contains a statement about the functional intent of the exercises.

O:   Veteran seen in room for AROM and strengthening of Ⓛ UE in order to regain ability to dress self. Pt. performed self-ranging exercises from standing and seated position with standby Ⓐ and verbal instructions to correct errors. Pt. was verbally cued x 5 to reach higher with Ⓛ UE during shoulder flexion AROM.

## Use Only Standard Abbreviations

You may use the abbreviations approved by your facility. For purposes of demonstration, a list of common abbreviations is provided in *Chapter 2: The Medical Record*. **Do not** use any other abbreviations, even if they seem common to you. If you try to read a note containing abbreviations with which you are unfamiliar, you will understand instantly how important this is. Remember that your documentation may be read by those unfamiliar with the shorthand that health professionals use so freely. Suppose your chart is being read by someone who is from a different background, such as an insurance clerk or an attorney or a committee at the Lions Club who is considering funding a piece of adaptive equipment for your patient. To make your note understandable to all its readers, be judicious in applying abbreviations and keep them very standard.

## Evaluation Notes

Many facilities have forms or checklists for recording evaluation data in order to make it quicker to document. There may be times, however, when you will record your evaluation in a SOAP format. There is additional information about requirements for different kinds of notes in *Chapter 10: Documenting Different Stages of Treatment.*

In an evaluation note, the "O" contains the data you collected in your evaluation including functional status and the results of any tests you might have performed to determine the limits of the performance components. It is best to assess function or performance areas first, followed by any performance components that may be interfering with those performance areas found not to be WFL.

For example:

O:  Pt. seen in room for initial evaluation including mini mental status exam.

*Dressing:* Skilled instruction on proper sitting position while dressing lower body and verbal cues to follow hip precautions. SBA required to insert arms into dress and pull down. Mod Ⓐ to place pad into underwear. Max. Ⓐ to pull underwear to hips; mod Ⓐ to waist. Max. Ⓐ to don shoes and socks due to hip precautions. Pt. needed verbal cues to follow hip precautions.

*Functional Mobility:* Verbal cues needed to stand using walker to follow hip precautions. Pt. requires min. Ⓐ sit ↔ stand.

*AROM:* UE: WFL

| Strength: | R | L |
|---|---|---|
| Ⓑ elbow flexion | 4- | 4- |
| Ⓑ elbow extension | 3+ | 3+ |
| Ⓑ shoulder flexion/extension | 3+ | 3+ |

*Cognition:* 28/30 on MMSE; O X 4; remembered 3 items.

## Discharge, Progress, and Reassessment Notes

Discharge, progress, and reassessment notes will also contain an amount of objective data. Usually a progress or reassessment summarizes a patient's progress to date, and a discharge note summarizes the patient's stay. This provides both a beginning and an ending picture of the patient's functional abilities.

O:    Pt. was referred to outpatient hand rehabilitation by Dr. Morris on 1/5/99. At that time she was unable to work and was receiving workman's compensation. She also reported difficulties caring for her family due to pain and stiffness in her hands. Pt. has been seen 3 x wk. for 1 hr. sessions to work on bilateral hand/wrist/finger strengthening, PROM and AROM since 1/5/98. In addition she has used a program of exercises 2 x daily at home.

Initial Pain 6/10
Initial Numbness Ⓡ 8/10 Ⓛ 10/10
9 Hole Peg:    Initial Ⓡ In: 10.6 Out: 4.7
               Initial Ⓛ In: 8.7 Out: 4.6

DC Pain 2/10
DC Numbness Ⓑ 0/10
DC In: 9.9 Out: 4.6
DC In: 8.1 Out: 4.0

Grip strength:
Initial (lbs)
Ⓡ 40,46,39,33,19
Ⓛ 30,47,35,38,21

DC (lbs)
Ⓡ 35,37,41,36,27
Ⓛ 40,54,47,38,31

Pinch:
Lateral (Key) (lbs)

| Initial | DC |
|---------|-----|
| Ⓡ 10 | 13½ |
| Ⓛ 9 | 16 |

3 Point (tip) (lbs)

| Initial | DC |
|---------|-----|
| Ⓡ 11 | 15 |
| Ⓛ 12½ | 14 |

When documenting test results, it is helpful to put the test results into a chart like the one above rather than burying them in a narrative. For example:

**Sensory testing of Ⓛ hand revealed:**
Hot/cold:      intact
Sharp/dull:    impaired over volar surface, intact over dorsal surface
Stereognosis:  absent

The "O" section does not need to be complete sentences. Give complete information in as concise a form as possible. Some details **must** be included. For example, ROM must be specified as active, passive, or assistive and must indicate the joint at which the movement occurred. UE must indicate which UE level of assistance must be specified if assistance was given.

# Common Errors

## Listing Only Assist Levels

When first learning to write the "O" section of the note, it is difficult to separate the objective data from the assessment data. Good therapists automatically assess the data as they observe. In trying to separate "O" data from "A" data, some therapists make the mistake of writing an "O" that contains only a list of actions with assist levels. While this is common, it is **incorrect**. A list of assist levels does not show skilled OT being provided. Consider this therapist's observation.

Pt. was seen in the shower room to ↑ activity tolerance and improve balance during showering, and was shown a smaller shower which simulated her home shower, in order to prepare for discharge in 1 week.
Pt. min Ⓐ with verbal cues to sit in w/c to doff hosiery and to dry off LE.
Pt. spontaneously rinsed soap off hands before grabbing grab bar while showering.
Pt. used walker going to/coming from shower room.
Pt. tolerated standing Ⓘ during entire shower.
Pt. instructed in home showering.

Now let us look at the same observation, rewritten in a more useful format.

> *Pt. was seen in the shower room to ↑ activity tolerance and improve balance during shower-ing and was also shown a smaller shower which simulated her home shower, in order to prepare her for ① and safe showering after discharge in 1 week.*

> **Cognition:** *Pt. oriented X 4.*

> **Mobility:** *Pt. walked to/from shower room ① and safely with the aid of a standard walker. Walker not necessary for patient's mobility, but rather for stability in shower room while dress-ing/undressing.*

> **ADL:** *Pt. min assist with verbal cues to sit down in order to towel dry LEs safely and to doff hosiery. During shower, pt. spontaneously rinsed soap off hands prior to gripping grab bar without verbal cues. Pt. tolerated standing ① during shower without SOB. Skilled instruction provided in safe technique to use in her single shower stall and recommendations given, re: grab bar placement.*

## Focusing on the Media

Another common error among new therapists is to focus on the media used, rather than on the performance component that is being improved by use of the media. Consider this therapist's observation.

> *Pt. was seen in rehab center for standing balance activities. Pt. stood to walker with min. Ⓐ for balloon toss with OTs. Pt. used Ⓡ UE to hit balloon and was able to reach to Ⓡ and Ⓛ sides approximately 7 out of 10 tries. Activity was continued for 3 minutes. Pt. requested rest break and sat for 30 seconds. Pt. then stood with mod Ⓐ to walker and hit balloon with Ⓛ UE for 3 minutes. Pt. was able to hit balloon approximately 6 out of 10 times and spon-taneously switched to Ⓡ hand x 2 when balloon was to her far right. Pt. sat for another break and to switch activities. Pt. stood CGA to toss bean bags with Ⓡ hand for 4 minutes. Pt. scored 240 points with Ⓡ hand by throwing bean bags at target. Once all bean bags were thrown, pt. sat for a 30-second break. Pt. stood with CGA to toss bean bags with Ⓛ hand for 30 sec-onds. Pt. scored 150 points with Ⓛ hand by throwing bean bags at scoring target. Once all bean bags were thrown, pt. sat and session was ended.*

When this note is rewritten to focus on the performance components, notice the difference in professionalism in the way the note reads.

> *Pt. seen in clinic for dynamic and static standing balance activities. Pt stood to walker with mod Ⓐ for dynamic standing balance necessary for ① showering using a balloon toss activ-ity. Pt. used Ⓡ UE to reach both Ⓡ and Ⓛ sides approximately 7/10 attempts. Pt. sustained activity for 3 minutes continuously and then took a 30-second rest break. Pt. stood to walker again with mod Ⓐ for 3 minutes of continuous activity involving weight shifting and balance required in balloon tossing. Pt. demonstrated ability to reach to Ⓡ and Ⓛ sides to reach for moving object approximately 6/10 times. Pt. demonstrated ability to spontaneously shift weight two times to reach object. Pt. took 30-second rest break before next activity. Pt. worked on dynamic standing balance using bean bag toss activity with target. Pt. stood to walker for 4 minutes of continuous light activity and sat for 30-second rest. Pt. stood again with CGA for 3½ minutes of continuous light activity.*

In mental health settings, it is particularly important to focus on the purpose of the activity if craft projects or other creative media is being used. For example, you may be using a creative proj-ect to facilitate *self-esteem*, to encourage *self-expression*, or to evaluate the ability to *follow instruc-tions*. This should be the focus of your note, rather than the project that was used.

# WORKSHEET 6-2

## Being Specific About Assist Levels

When noting assist levels in your observation, it is not enough to note just the level of assistance required. You also need to note the **part** of the task that required assistance.

For example:

*Pt. donned pants with min.* Ⓐ *to pull up over hips.*

*Pt. propelled W/C from room to OT clinic but required verbal cues **to avoid running into other patients**.*

Assistance to sequence an activity is very different from assistance to maintain balance or to reach the feet while observing hip precautions.

**Rewrite the statements below to provide a part of the task that required assistance.**

1.    Pt. supine → sit with min Ⓐ , bed → w/c with mod Ⓐ.

2.    Pt. required SBA in transferring w/c ⇆ toilet.

3.    Pt. retrieved garments from low drawers with min Ⓐ.

4.    Brushing hair required max Ⓐ.

5.    Pt. completed dressing, toileting, and hygiene with min Ⓐ.

*From Borcherding S. Documentation Manual for Writing SOAP Notes in Occupational Therapy.* © 2000 SLACK Incorporated

# Deemphasizing the Treatment Media

When writing about what you observe, one of the most obvious items you may see is the media used. Consider the way this therapist has chosen to document her observation of what the patient did.

*Patient worked on placing pegs into a pegboard.*

On the surface this seems accurate, and it may in fact be what a casual observer would see. As a trained professional you will look beyond the media used such as the pegboard to observe what the patient was really working on. What is the performance component here? Placing pegs into a pegboard is not a skill this patient needs in order to be able to care for herself. The performance component she is practicing may well be important to her independence. Suppose the therapist had written the following:

*Patient worked on tripod pinch using pegs and a pegboard.*

Notice that in this example the therapist did not simply add the performance component to the statement, but actually turned the sentence around so that the tripod pinch that the patient was actually doing received the emphasis and the media was mentioned only for clarification. Suppose that the therapist had written:

*Patient worked on tripod pinch in order to be able to grasp objects needed for ADL tasks.*

In this case, mention of the media becomes optional. She could also have written:

*Patient worked on tripod pinch using pegs and a pegboard in order to be able to grasp objects needed for ADL tasks.*

Which of the three preceding examples do you think best describes the skilled instruction that is occurring in this treatment session? This may seem like a minor distinction, but it is a very important one.

# WORKSHEET 6-3

## *Deemphasizing the Treatment Media*

Rewrite the following statements to emphasize the skilled OT that is actually occurring in the treatment session.

1.  Patient played pegboard game to work on functional grasp.

2.  Patient played catch using bilateral UEs to facilitate grasp and release pattern.

3.  Patient put dirt into pot to ½ way point, added seedling, and filled remainder of pot with dirt transferred by cup. Pt. completed 3 more pots while standing 8 minutes before requiring a 5-minute rest. Pt. resumed standing position to water completed pots for approximately 5 minutes.

The treatment media also needs to be deemphasized in writing goal statements. Rewrite these two goal statements to focus on the performance area and performance components rather than on the media.

1.  Patient will place 8 ½ inch screws and washers on a block of wood with holes while sitting by 4/10/98.

2.  Pt. will make a clock using the appropriate materials while sitting by discharge.

# CHAPTER 7
## Writing the "A"—Assessment

The third section of the note is the **Assessment** in which the therapist reports his or her professional opinions and judgments as to the patient's functional limitations and expected benefit from rehabilitation.

## Evaluation Note

In an **evaluation note**, the assessment section will contain the problem list and the rehabilitation potential of the patient.

> *A:*     *Deficits noted in Ⓡ UE A/PROM and strength which limit ability to perform self-care skills, e.g., dressing, grooming, hygiene, toileting. Deficits also noted in dynamic balance, which impacts safety during transfers and standing. Pt. has difficulty with receptive and expressive language, with following one stage commands, and orientation, making her unsafe in home management tasks. Pt. exhibits intact body awareness and there is no evidence of Ⓡ unilateral neglect. Pt. would benefit from activities to increase A/PROM and strength in Ⓡ UE, increase Ⓘ in self-care skills, increase safety during transfers, increase standing activity tolerance. She would also benefit from orientation to the environment. Rehab potential is good for return to home.*

## Treatment Note

In the assessment section of a **treatment note**, you will assess the meaning of the data presented in the "O" portion of the note. Describe what it means in your professional judgment. In the assessment section you may also point out inconsistencies, justify your goals, discuss emotional status, point out patient's strengths, indicate progress in therapy, or discuss rehabilitation potential. You may present reasons some information was not obtained, recommend further testing or treatment that you think is necessary, or suggest a referral to another professional or to a community service. This is your opportunity to draw conclusions from the other parts of the note that may not be obvious to others.

> *A:*     *Inability to don prosthesis Ⓘ currently limits Ⓘ in ambulation/functional toileting. Pt. would benefit from additional skilled instruction in use of pulley-like fasteners on prosthesis to manage one-handed closure installed this date.*

> *A:*     *Martha is beginning to regain some of the independent living skills she had prior to her recent psychotic episode. Fear, isolation, and ↓ activity tolerance slow her progress and are the focus of current treatment. Martha would benefit from continued skilled instruction in self-care skills as well as ↑ socialization and ↑ physical activity.*

> *A:*     *Mary uses her Ⓛ hand as a functional assist 60% of the time, which continues to limit her Ⓘ in self-care and play tasks. She would benefit from more Ⓑ activities to ↑ use of Ⓛ hand during play.*

## Assessing the Data

To assess the data, go **sentence by sentence** through the data presented in the "O," asking yourself what it means for the patient's occupational performance. Consider some of the following possibilities.

Evidence that the treatment provided was effective. For example:

*Weighted utensils ↓ intention tremors by ~ 50%.*

Evidence of patient progress or explanation of failure to progress as quickly as anticipated. For example:

*Patient has gained 10° active range of motion in the ⒧ elbow since last treatment session.*

*Patient has made gains since 11/17/98 by demonstrating the ability to follow 1-step commands 80% of the time.*

*Patient has become more Ⓓ in ADL tasks this week due to fatigue 2° acute infection.*

*Patient responded positively to instructions in self-care activities and adaptations by expressing her desire to be Ⓘ .*

Inconsistencies between patient report and objective findings. For example:

*Although patient anticipates no difficulty in returning to pre-hospitalization level of home-making activity, her left side neglect could cause significant in-home safety risks.*

*Although patient expresses a willingness to do ADLs, motor planning problems create a barrier to the task.*

*Although resident requests help learning to don and doff shoes Ⓘ , decreased vision and decreased LE AROM make prognosis for total Ⓘ in donning/doffing shoes guarded.*

Evidence of safety risks. For example:

*Safety concerns noted when patient attempted to stand without locking brakes on w/c.*

*Patient problem-solved poorly while using the stove, posing safety concerns.*

Areas of performance not WFL that can be influenced by OT intervention. For example:

*Problem areas include completing sit→stand without assistance, decreased flexibility in LE, reduced dressing activity tolerance, and inability to fasten buttons on shirt.*

*Pt. showed some delayed cognitive processing requiring instructions to be repeated 3 times.*

*Patient displayed left UE visual/tactile inattention, left UE sensory deficits, slowed cognition, and decreased motor planning.*

*Left side weakness interferes with standing balance in tub.*

*Patient demonstrates left side neglect, needing verbal cues to complete ADLs.*

*Due to cognitive problems, patient currently needs constant verbal cues to perform all ADL tasks.*

## New Information

The assessment section is **not** the place to introduce new data. Do not put anything in your "A" that has not been discussed in "O." If you find yourself wanting to make a statement in the "A" that is not supported by the data in your "O," ask yourself what you might have observed to support the assessment statement. Then decide whether you need to add it to your "O."

## Justifying Continued Treatment

One very useful way of justifying continued skilled OT for your patient is to end the "A" with the statement "Patient would benefit from..." and complete the sentence with a justification of continued skilled OT, based on your observations and assessment. Not every therapist ends the "A" in this fashion, but for purposes of learning this is the way we will end the "A." This helps to make certain that justification for continued treatment is present in the note, and is a good method of setting up the plan. After you are more proficient in writing notes and are certain that your note justifies continued treatment, you may choose to cover this material in the plan instead.

*Patient would benefit from cues to orient him to environment.*

*Patient would benefit from further ADL training along with visual, perceptual, and problem-solving activities.*

*Patient would benefit from activities that encourage trunk rotation to facilitate Ⓘ in transfers and dressing skills.*

*Patient would benefit from reacher, sock aid, and long-handled shoe horn to aid in LE dressing.*

*Patient would benefit from skilled instruction in sequencing of tasks to increase safety while performing ADL tasks.*

*Patient would benefit from instruction in energy conservation techniques to perform meal preparation and cleanup.*

In addition, it is necessary to document the reason the service must be provided by an OTR or COTA rather than by another professional or by nonprofessional personnel.

Registered occupational therapists provide the following services:
- Evaluate patients, identify problems, establish goals, and develop treatment plans
- Assess or reassess the effectiveness of adaptive equipment/techniques

Registered occupational therapists and certified occupational therapy assistants provide the following services:
- Modify functional tasks/activities, modify homes, or other environmental contexts
- Modify activities through the use of adaptive equipment/assistive devices
- Provide and instruct in the use of adaptive equipment; instruct in adaptive techniques
- Fabricate splints and adaptive devices
- Provide individualized instruction to the patient/family/caregiver
- Determine that the procedure/equipment used is safe and effective
- Intervene to prevent safety hazards and unsafe behaviors
- Teach compensatory skills
- Improve performance areas through remediation approaches
- Instruct in energy conservation and work simplification
- Instruct in joint protection (Cullen, 1998).

Skilled occupational therapy is NOT evident when the OTR or COTA:

- Continues treatment after goals are reached or no further significant progress is expected
- Carries out a maintenance program
- Provides routine strengthening or exercise programs if there is no potential for functional improvement
- Carries out daily programs after the adapted procedures are in place and no further progress is expected
- Presents information such as handouts on energy conservation without having the patient or caregiver perform the activity
- Provides service to a patient who has poor rehabilitation potential
- Duplicates services with another discipline (Cullen, 1998)

Wording is critical to documenting the necessity for continuing skilled occupational therapy. For example, occupational therapy personnel **provide skilled instruction** to patients rather than assisting them. Occupational therapists **design** home programs that may be **carried out** by aides or family members.

Why should a third party payer reimburse you to watch a patient carry out his home exercise program that he performs daily on his own? However, if you are **evaluating** his ability to do all the components of it correctly, or **modifying** it to compensate for recent progress, then your professional skill is clearly required. Analyze your clinical reasoning and then document the principles and strategies used during a treatment session in justifying the continuation of skilled occupational therapy.

Remember that the assessment and the justification for continued skilled OT must support the frequency and duration of the plan. If the last sentence of your "A" reads *patient would benefit from information on energy conservation techniques*, do not expect to have a plan approved for more than one more treatment session.

If this is your last session, complete the sentence with your discharge plan. For example:

*Patient would benefit from continued PROM provided by restorative aide.*

*Patient has been instructed in home exercise program and has demonstrated ability to perform correctly.*

*Patient would benefit from adaptations to the home.*

---

**HELPFUL HINT**

Assessment is the "heart" of your note. If you could write only six lines, the assessment section of your note would contain the six lines you would choose. This is the section that demonstrates your clinical reasoning as an occupational therapist.

# WORKSHEET 7-1

## Justifying Skilled Occupational Therapy

**Which of the following meet the criterion for skilled occupational therapy?**

_____ Evaluation of a patient

_____ The practice of coordination and self-care skills on a daily basis

_____ Establishing measurable, behavioral, objective, and individualized goals

_____ Developing treatment plans that are designed to meet the established goals

_____ Carrying out a maintenance program

_____ Analyzing and modifying functional tasks/activities through the provision of adaptive equipment or techniques

_____ Determining that the modified task is safe and effective

_____ Carrying a breathing retraining program into ADL training

_____ Providing individualized instruction to the patient, family, or caregiver

_____ Reevaluating the patient's status

_____ Modifying the treatment plan based on the reevaluation

_____ Provision of specialized instruction to eliminate limitations in a functional activity

_____ Developing a home program and instructing caregivers

_____ Making changes in the environment

_____ Teaching compensatory skills

_____ Gait training

_____ Intervening with patients to eliminate safety hazards

_____ Presenting information handouts (such as energy conservation) without having the patient perform the activity

_____ Routine exercise and strengthening programs

_____ Preparing a problem list which identifies present status and potential capabilities

_____ Adding teaching lower body dressing to a current program

_____ Teaching adaptive techniques such as one-handed shoe tying

# An Observation Using Categories

In *Chapter 5, Writing the "S"—Subjective*, the following observation was used as a demonstration. Now we will look at its content more carefully, look at the suggestions given earlier in this chapter, and draw some conclusions.

**S:** *Patient says she is unable to move right UE, although she does not know why it will not move. She reports, "It really doesn't hurt. It's just tight."*

**O:** *Patient seen in rehab gym for UE activities to ↑ AROM in ⓇR shoulder, activity tolerance, UE strength, and dynamic standing balance, in order to ↑ independence in ADL activities.*

***ADL:*** *Pt. seen in room for instruction in safety techniques and adaptive equipment use in toileting. Pt. needs bilateral grab bars in bathroom to sit ⇆ stand safely. Pt. attempted to stand while pulling on walker and one grab bar. Pt. was instructed on safety issues and the use of bilateral grab bars.*

***Performance Components:*** *Pt. sit → stand CGA for balance. Pt. worked on activity tolerance, dynamic standing balance, and ↑AROM in ⓇR shoulder by moving canned goods from counter to cupboard for 5 minutes before needing a 2-minute sitting rest. After resting, she poured liquid from a pitcher while standing CGA for balance. After 1-minute rest, pt. pushed wheeled walker while picking up objects from the floor with a reacher in order to increase dynamic standing balance and safety in ADL activities. AROM in right shoulder abduction <90°. PROM right shoulder abduction WNL.*

**How would you assess this information? Do you see evidence of progress? Safety risks? Performance areas not WFL that occupational therapy might impact? What would this patient benefit from? Write your "A" assessment based on the information above.**

# Assessing the Categories Note

In preparing an assessment of the data in this note, this therapist assesses the safety both of transferring to and from the toilet, and the performance components. This therapist was particularly concerned about the safety issues, and addressed them first.

> *A:*      *Safety concerns noted when patient attempts to transfer sit ⇆ stand during toileting. Pt. seemed to understand safety instructions and has potential to progress to Ⓘ.*

She also noted the rehabilitation potential that would be helpful to a reviewer in deciding whether the patient's progress is sufficient to warrant the expense of treatment.

Next she addressed the clinical reasoning behind devoting time to addressing performance components with this patient, in light of his rehab potential.

> *A:*      *Safety concerns noted when patient attempts to transfer sit ⇆ stand during toileting. Pt. seemed to understand safety instructions and has potential to progress to Ⓘ. Pt.'s ↓ AROM Ⓡ shoulder, ↓ activity tolerance, and ↓ dynamic standing balance all interfere with ability to complete ADLs safely and independently.*

She completes the assessment by justifying continued skilled occupational therapy.

> *A:*      *Safety concerns (impulsivity, ↓ dynamic standing balance) noted when patient attempts to transfer sit ⇆ stand during toileting. Pt. seemed to understand safety instructions and has potential to progress to Ⓘ. Pt.'s ↓ AROM Ⓡ shoulder, ↓activity tolerance, and ↓ dynamic standing balance all interfere with ability to complete ADLs safely and independently. Pt. would benefit from UE AROM and strengthening exercises along with continued skilled instruction in safety issues and energy conservation techniques.*

In *Chapter 8, Writing the "P"—Plan,* you will see how this therapist specifies how to provide this recommended treatment in a cost-effective manner.

# CHAPTER 8
## Writing the "P"—Plan

The last section of a SOAP note is the **Plan** where the therapist sets forth the specific treatment that the patient will receive to achieve the goals. The plan should relate to the information you have just presented. It will inform the reader what you plan to do next in treatment, and should include your long- or short-term goals.

## Initial Evaluation Report

In an **initial evaluation report** this section will contain both the long- and short-term goals, as well as the frequency and duration of treatment.

## Treatment Notes

For the purpose of **treatment notes**, you will address any part of your plan for this patient that has not been covered above, such as how often and/or how long you plan to continue treatment. End with either your long-term goal or your short-term goal, whichever is appropriate to your treatment setting. (Usually the short-term goal is used.) Goals are always written in measurable, objective, behavioral terms, and include a function and a time line. For example:

Pt. will _____ _____ _____
        *Action verb*         *Skill*         *Under what conditions*

_____ _____.
  *For what function—if not already indicated*         *By when*

Examples of a "P" might include:

*Resident to be seen for 2 more weeks for ½ hr. b.i.d. sessions for skilled instruction in meal/snack preparation and clean up. By discharge on 8/13/99, resident will be able to prepare a TV dinner in the microwave Ⓘ at wheelchair level.*

*Continue 1 hour daily sessions for 1 week. Within 1 week, veteran will demonstrate the ability to put arms in holes of shirt after set up and < 3 verbal cues 50% of the time.*

*Child to be seen 2 x wk for ½ hour sessions in order to ↑ fine motor skills for better classroom performance. Student will be able to cut a curved line with 75% accuracy 3/3 tries.*

*Pt. to be seen in groups 5 x wk for 1 week to work on assertion skills and anger management. Pt will attend 75% of groups without prompting and will spontaneously participate in discussion > 5 times by 4/2/99.*

*Consumer will continue sheltered workshop program 5 days/wk. in order to ↑ work skills. Consumer will attend to task for 60 minutes with no verbal cues within 1 week in order to ↑ Ⓘ as a worker.*

> **HELPFUL HINT**
> If for some reason you are not able to see your patient as scheduled, the "plan" section of your note should allow another therapist to continue treatment uninterrupted.

# Planning for the Categories Note

Now let us write a plan for the "Categories" note we assessed in the last chapter.

> S: Patient says she is unable to move right UE, although she does not know why it will not move. She reports, "It really doesn't hurt. It's just tight."

> O: Patient seen in rehab clinic for UE activities to ↑ AROM in Ⓡ shoulder, activity tolerance, UE strength, and dynamic standing balance, in order to ↑ independence in ADL tasks.

**ADL:** Pt. seen in room for instruction in safety techniques and adaptive equipment use in toileting. Pt. needs bilateral grab bars in bathroom to sit ⇆ stand safely. Patient attempted to stand while pulling on walker and one grab bar. Patient was instructed on safety issues and the use of bilateral grab bars.

**Performance components:** Pt. sit → stand CGA for balance. Pt. worked on activity tolerance, dynamic standing balance and ↑ AROM in Ⓡ shoulder by moving canned goods from counter to cupboard for 5 minutes before needing a 2-minute sitting rest. After resting, she poured liquid from a pitcher while standing CGA for balance. After 1-minute rest, pt. pushed wheeled walker while picking up objects from the floor with a reacher in order to increase dynamic standing balance and safety in ADL activities. AROM in right shoulder abduction <90°. PROM right shoulder abduction WNL.

> A: Safety concerns (impulsivity, ↓ dynamic standing balance) noted when patient attempts to transfer sit ⇆ stand during toileting. Pt. seemed to understand safety instructions and has potential to progress to Ⓘ. Pt.'s ↓ AROM Ⓡ shoulder, ↓ activity tolerance, and ↓ dynamic standing balance interfere with ability to complete ADLs safely and independently. Pt. would benefit from UE AROM and strengthening exercises along with continued skilled instruction in safety issues and energy conservation techniques.

**Write your plan for this patient below. Include how often and for how long you will want to see her as well as anything you might not have mentioned in "Pt. would benefit from..." End with either an STG or LTG goal.**

# Completing the Plan for the Categories Note

In assessing the data, the therapist has set up the plan for this note. She has already justified the main things she intended to do and indicated the patient's rehabilitation potential. Now she needs to be specific about how often she wants to treat the patient and for what length of time. She first specifies the frequency and duration of treatment.

> *P:*      *Patient will be seen 5 x wk. for 1 week.*

She could have specified the length of the treatment sessions, e.g., for 1 hr. sessions, but this therapist chose not to do that in this particular note. Next she specifies how she plans to use the treatment time.

> *P:*      *Patient will be seen 5 x wk. for 1 week for skilled instruction in safe transfers and toileting.*

Since she anticipates discharge in 1 week, she has to prioritize her time. She chooses to work on balance and energy conservation as a part of functional mobility and ADL activities. Since she has already written that the patient would benefit from additional AROM and strengthening exercises, she now needs to specify how she plans to address this need.

> *P:*      *Patient will be seen 5 x wk. for 1 week for skilled instruction in safe transfers and toileting. Home program for AROM and strengthening exercises for Ⓡ shoulder will be taught.*

This therapist has also indicated her clinical reasoning in planning for discharge in advance of the discharge date. In later notes she will indicate the patient's progress in learning the home program. Simply handing the patient a set of printed exercises is not considered a billable service. The patient's progress in learning the home program will also confirm the therapist's assessment that the patient's rehabilitation potential was on target. She will end this plan with a measurable, action oriented, time-limited goal. Notice that she has specified the conditions under which this action will be carried out.

> *P:*      *Patient will be seen 5 x wk. for 1 week to work on safe transfers and toileting. Home program for AROM and strengthening exercises for Ⓡ shoulder will be taught. Pt. will demonstrate ability to transfer to toilet safely with CGA and use of walker and grab bars by the end of 5 tx. sessions.*

This note is now complete.

# Final SOAP Note for a Treatment Session Written in Categories

> *S:*      *Pt. says she is unable to move right UE, although she does not know why it will not move. She reports, "It really doesn't hurt. It's just tight."*
>
> *O:*      *Pt. seen in rehab gym for UE activities to ↑ AROM in Ⓡ shoulder, activity tolerance, UE strength, and dynamic standing balance in order to ↑ independence in ADL activities.*
>
> *ADL: Pt. seen in room for instruction in safety techniques and adaptive equipment use in toileting. Pt. needs bilateral grab bars in bathroom to sit ⇆ stand safely. Pt. attempted to stand while pulling on walker and one grab bar. Pt. was instructed on safety issues and the use of bilateral grab bars.*

*Performance components:* Pt. sit → stand CGA for balance. Pt. worked on activity tolerance, dynamic standing balance and ↑ AROM in ⓡ shoulder by moving canned goods from counter to cupboard for 5 minutes before needing a 2-minute sitting rest. After resting, she poured liquid from a pitcher while standing CGA for balance. After 1-minute rest, pt. pushed wheeled walker while picking up objects from the floor with a reacher in order to increase dynamic standing balance and safety in ADL activities. AROM in right shoulder abduction < 90°. PROM right shoulder abduction WNL.

**A:**  Safety concerns (impulsivity, ↓ dynamic standing balance) noted when patient attempts to transfer sit ⇆ stand during toileting. Pt. seemed to understand safety instructions and has potential to progress to ⓘ. Pt.'s ↑ AROM ⓡ shoulder, ↓ activity tolerance, and ↓ dynamic standing balance all interfere with ability to complete ADLs safely and independently. Pt. would benefit from UE AROM and strengthening exercises along with continued skilled instruction in safety issues and energy conservation techniques.

**P:**  Patient will be seen 5 x wk. for 1 week for skilled instruction in safe transfers and toileting. Home program for AROM and strengthening exercises for ⓡ shoulder will be taught. Pt. will demonstrate ability to transfer to toilet safely with CGA and use of walker and grab bars by the end of 5 tx. sessions.

Tara Grantham, OTR/L

# Observation of a Treatment Session
# Primarily Devoted to Exercise

Read the following observation of a treatment session and formulate an assessment and a plan based on the information provided. Please do not read ahead to find out how the therapist writing the note words the "A" and "P" sections. It is far more effective to test your skill at writing assessments and plans before finding out how someone else might have written the same information.

S:  *Pt. reports being pleased with her progress in functional mobility since last tx. session.*

O:  *Pt. was seen in OT clinic to work on bilateral UE strengthening and AROM in order to improve bilateral UE function in ADLs. She required min assist with w/c mobility room → clinic, requiring verbal instructions not to hit the wall and an occasional push when she lost momentum.*

*Pt. then completed left UE strengthening exercises using yellow Thera-Band (The Hygenic Corporation, Akron, Ohio):*
   *elbow flexion x 15*
   *elbow extension x 15*

*Pt. then completed right UE strengthening and AROM with the following results:*
   *right forearm: pronation: full AROM supination: ½ AROM*
   *right wrist: extension: ½ AROM (x10 repetitions)*
   *radial and ulnar deviation: WFL*
   *fingers: flexion and extension: full AROM*
   *thumb: opposition: full AROM*

*Pt. was able to demonstrate isolated 3+ finger flexion and extension in all five digits against no resistance. Brunnstrom arm exercises with AAROM to right UE to increase strength and AROM for donning shirt using over the head method.*

*Results: (bilateral shoulder)*
   *elevation/depression x 5*
   *flexion x 5*
   *horizontal ab/adduction x 5*

**Write your "A" assessment and "P" plan below.**

# Assessing and Planning for the Exercise Note

When a treatment session is devoted primarily to addressing performance components, it is critical to tie the performance components back into function. This note addresses function in some manner in all four sections, even though the treatment session was devoted to exercise. Note that in the observation, the therapist specified that the exercises were for the purpose of improving UE function in ADL tasks. In the assessment she will reiterate that she is basically trying to improve function in ADL tasks by working on the underlying factors that prevent independent functioning.

Having reported the basic measurements and assist levels in the "O," the therapist interprets the meaning of these in her assessment.

> **A:**     *Patient demonstrates improved w/c mobility from mod Ⓐ last Thursday to min Ⓐ today. Pt. also demonstrates ↑ AROM in all 5 digits and ↑ activity tolerance in wrist extension (x 10 repetitions) from last Thursday (x 5 repetitions).*

This therapist basically plans to continue with the same program since she is seeing good progress.

> **A:**     *Patient demonstrates improved w/c mobility from mod Ⓐ last Thursday to min Ⓐ today. Pt. also demonstrates ↑ AROM in all 5 digits and ↑ activity tolerance in wrist extension (x 10) from last Thursday (x 5). Pt. would benefit from further strengthening and AROM to reach the 4+ UE strength and 3/4 AROM needed for independence in ADL tasks.*

A program of routine exercises is not billable as skilled occupational therapy. Therefore, this therapist has shifted the responsibility for the exercise program to an aide because she has determined what kind of exercise program the patient needed.

> **P:**     *Continue Ⓑ UE exercises daily for 1 wk. under supervision of an aide to ↑ strength, activity tolerance, and AROM.*

She plans to continue seeing the patient and to use the treatment sessions to accomplish the other goals that require the skill of an occupational therapist. The goal she establishes is related to the sessions she will carry out based on the performance components that are being addressed by the aide.

> **P:**     *Continue Ⓑ UE exercises daily for 1 wk. under supervision of an aide to ↑ strength, activity tolerance, and AROM. Skilled OT 3 x wk. for work on specific ADL tasks of dressing, grooming, hygiene @ 1 hr./visit.*

She ends the note with the short-term goal.

> **P:**     *Continue Ⓑ UE exercises daily for 1 wk. under supervision of an aide to ↑ strength, activity tolerance, and AROM. Skilled OT 3 x wk. for work on specific ADL tasks of dressing, bathing, grooming @ 1 hr./visit. Pt. will be Ⓘ in ADL tasks by discharge in 2 weeks.*

# SOAP Note for a Treatment Session Primarily Devoted to Exercise

**S:** Pt. reports being pleased with her progress in functional mobility since last tx. session.

**O:** Pt. was seen in OT clinic to work on bilateral UE strengthening and AROM in order to improve bilateral UE function in ADL tasks. She required min assist with w/c mobility room→clinic, requiring verbal instructions not to hit the wall and an occasional push when she lost momentum. Pt. then completed left UE strengthening exercises using yellow Thera-Band:

> elbow flexion x 15
> elbow extension x 15

Pt. then completed right UE strengthening and AROM with the following results:

> right forearm: pronation: full AROM; supination: ½ AROM
> right wrist: extension: ½ AROM (x 10 repetitions)
> radial and ulnar deviation: WFL
> fingers: flexion and extension: full AROM
> thumb: opposition: full AROM

Pt. was able to demonstrate isolated 3+ finger flexion and extension in all five digits against no resistance. Brunnstrom arm exercises with AAROM to right UE to increase strength and AROM for donning shirt using over the head method. Results: (bilateral shoulder)

> elevation/depression x 5
> flexion x 5
> horizontal ab/adduction  x 5

**A:** Pt. demonstrates improved w/c mobility from mod Ⓐ last Thursday to min Ⓐ today. Pt. also demonstrates ↑ AROM in all 5 digits and ↑ activity tolerance in wrist extension (x 10) from last Thursday (x 5). Pt. would benefit from further strengthening and AROM to reach the 4+ UE strength and 3/4 AROM needed for independence in ADL tasks.

**P:** Continue Ⓑ UE exercises daily for 1 wk. under supervision of an aide to ↑ strength, activity tolerance, and AROM. Skilled OT 3 x wk. for work on specific ADL tasks of dressing, bathing, grooming @ 1 hr./visit. Pt. will be Ⓘ in ADLs by discharge in 2 weeks.

Heather Yamnitz, OTR/L

# Observation of a One-Visit-Only Treatment Session

**S:**     *Pt. reports that 2 to 3 weeks after car accident in December of 1997 she began experiencing numbness in digits 1, 2, and 3 of her dominant right hand. During the evaluation she reported tingling in her right hand while performing strengthening exercises. She also stated that she carried her infant primarily on the right side.*

**O:**     *Pt. seen in OT outpatient clinic for assessment and educational activities to improve functional activities in right hand. Results of evaluation are as follows:*
*Manual muscle test of right wrist:  extension 3/5; flexion 4/5; pronation/supination 4/5*
*Grip strength: Right: 56, 60, 85, 81, 65        Left: 39, 75, 75, 73, 59*
*Pinch: Lateral: 19 right 17½ left               Tripod: 15 right 12.5 left*
*Edema: mild*
*Volumeter: Right: 1500 ml water displacement   Left: 1470 ml water displacement*
*9 Hole Peg Test: 35 right 39 left*

*Pt. instructed in and performed strengthening exercises for right UE, 15 repetitions for each, all AROM through full range:*
*wrist extension using a 1 lb weight*
*radial/ulnar deviation using a 2 lb weight*
*pronation/supination using a 24 oz. weight on hammer*

*Pt. instructed to squeeze a soft or wet washcloth and theraputty daily, and to interchange carrying baby on left as well as on right arm.*

*Pt. instructed in and performed finger abduction/adduction exercises with a rubberband for right hand with fingers in slight (10°) flexion. Pt. instructed to use 2 rubber bands at a time and to perform 3 to 4 times daily at home. Pt. was instructed in and performed hand strengthening exercises 15 repetitions through full AROM.*
*wrist extension using a 1 lb weight*
*radial/ulnar deviation using a 2 lb weight*
*pronation/supination using a 24 oz. weight on hammer*

*Pt. instructed to squeeze a soft or wet washcloth and theraputty daily, and to interchange carrying baby on left as well as on right arm.*

*Pt. instructed in and performed finger abduction/adduction exercises with a rubberband for right hand with fingers in slight (10°) flexion. Pt. instructed to use 2 rubberbands at a time and to perform 3 to 4 times daily at home. Pt. was instructed in and performed hand strengthening exercises 15 repetitions through full AROM. Pt. fitted with orthoplast volar cockup splint and instructed to wear at bedtime. Pt. instructed in edema management and correct positioning to avoid stress to carpal tunnel structure. Pt. given written handout of exercises and demonstrated under standing by performing each correctly.*

**Write your "A" assessment and "P" plan for this note below.**

# Assessing and Planning for the One-Visit-Only Note

This note is a little different, because it is a one-time visit. The therapist had to evaluate, treat, and discharge the patient all in one session. The therapist has chosen to be brief in her assessment of this data, stating what the patient reported and what the evaluation showed, and indicating that it interfered with function.

> A:  ↑ numbness in digits 1,2, & 3 in combination with ↓ bilateral coordination as noted on the 9 hole peg test and ↑ Ⓡ UE edema interfere with ability to perform ADL tasks.

This is a one-time-only treatment session and the therapist did not use the assessment and planning section to make a problem list and indicate rehabilitation potential. **If this patient were to be followed in outpatient OT over the course of several weeks, the therapist would need to be more detailed in her assessment of the evaluation data.** She wonders whether she might be seeing the beginning of carpal tunnel syndrome, but isn't able to address it very well in one visit with the other treatment she has to accomplish. Instead, she has included the component of prevention by providing instruction in positioning as a part of the exercise program.

The next statement might seem like an observation.

> Pt. verbalized understanding of home exercise program and was able to demonstrate exercises performed properly.

In this note, however, the therapist has explained in her "O" data that a home exercise program was given, and has explained exactly what the patient is to do. Now, in the "A", she makes the assessment that the patient is able to understand the HEP, as demonstrated by verbal statements and by performing the exercises correctly.

> A:  ↑ numbness in digits 1,2, & 3 in combination with ↓ bilateral coordination as noted on the 9 hole peg test and ↑ Ⓡ UE edema interfere with ability to perform ADL tasks. Pt. verbalized understanding of home exercise program and was able to demonstrate exercises performed properly.

Even though she will not see the patient again, she still indicates that the patient will benefit from this HEP and ties it to function.

> A:  ↑ numbness in digits 1 ,2, & 3 in combination with ↓ bilateral coordination as noted on the 9 hole peg test and ↑ Ⓡ UE edema interfere with ability to perform ADL tasks. Pt. verbalized understanding of home exercise program and was able to demonstrate exercises performed properly. Pt would benefit from further AROM and strengthening exercises to Ⓡ hand in order to ↓ inflammation and numbness and to ↑ functional performance of ADL tasks.

In her "P" plan, the therapist notes that it is a one-time visit and includes a note of the goals for this visit. The patient is discharged.

# SOAP Note for a One-Session-Only Treatment Session

> S:  Pt. reports that 2 to 3 weeks after car accident in December of 1997 she began experiencing numbness in digits 1, 2, & 3 of her dominant right hand. During the evaluation she reported tingling in her right hand while performing strengthening exercises. She also stated that she carried her infant primarily on the right side.

O:     *Pt. seen in OT outpatient clinic for assessment and educational activities to improve functional activities in right hand. Results of evaluation are as follows:*

*Manual muscle test of right wrist: extension 3/5; flexion 4/5; pronation/supination 4/5*

    *Grip strength: Right: 56, 60, 85, 81, 65        Left: 39, 75, 75, 73, 59*

    *Pinch: Lateral: 19 right 17½ left          Tripod: 15 right 12½ left*

    *Edema:        mild*

    *Volumeter: Right: 1500 ml water displacement    Left: 1470 ml water displacement*

    *9 Hole Peg Test: 35 right 39 left*

*Pt. instructed in and performed strengthening exercises for right UE, 15 repetitions for each, all AROM through full range:*

        *wrist extension using a 1 lb weight*

        *radial/ulnar deviation using a 2 lb weight*

        *pronation/supination using a 24 oz. weight on hammer*

*Pt. instructed to squeeze a soft or wet washcloth and putty daily, and to interchange carrying baby on left as well as on right arm.*

*Pt. instructed in and performed finger abduction/adduction exercises with a rubberband for right hand with fingers in slight (10°) flexion. Pt. instructed to use 2 rubber bands at a time and to perform 3 to 4 times daily at home. Pt. was instructed in and performed hand strengthening exercises 15 repetitions through full AROM.*

        *wrist extension using a 1 lb weight*

        *radial/ulnar deviation using a 2 lb weight*

        *pronation/supination using a 24 oz. weight on hammer*

*Pt. instructed to squeeze a soft or wet washcloth and putty daily, and to interchange carrying baby on left as well as on right arm.*

*Pt. instructed in and performed finger abduction/adduction exercises with a rubber band for right hand with fingers in slight (10°) flexion. Pt. instructed to use 2 rubber bands at a time and to perform 3 to 4 times daily at home. Pt. was instructed in and performed hand strengthening exercises 15 repetitions through full AROM. Pt. fitted with orthoplast volar cockup splint and instructed to wear at bedtime. Pt. instructed in edema management and correct positioning to avoid stress to carpal tunnel structure. Pt. given written handout of exercises and demonstrated understanding by performing each correctly.*

A:     *↑ numbness in digits 1, 2, and 3 in combination with ↓ bilateral coordination as noted on the 9 hole peg test and ↑ Ⓡ UE edema interfere with ability to perform ADL tasks. Pt. verbalized understanding of home exercise program and was able to demonstrate exercises performed properly. Pt would benefit from further AROM and strengthening exercises to Ⓡ hand in order to ↓ inflammation and numbness and to ↑ functional performance of ADL tasks.*

P:     *Pt. seen one time only per physician's order. Pt. to continue home exercise program.*

       *STG #1: Patient will demonstrate ability to perform strengthening exercises Ⓘ for Ⓡ hand after skilled instruction.*

       *STG #2: Patient will verbalize understanding of splint care and daily splint wearing schedule after skilled instruction.*

       *Pt. discharged having met both STGs this session.*

Marilyn Sunde, OTR/L

# WORKSHEET 8-1

## A Treatment Session Devoted to ADL Activities

S:      *Resident asked for help toileting. He responded to being addressed by name and indicated that it was time for his therapy. He was able to indicate the date and the time of day using a clock and calendar.*

O:      *Resident seen in room to work on dressing and toileting activities. Resident required verbal, written, and tactile cues throughout the session to maintain balance. When sitting on edge of bed patient was dependent in donning underwear and coveralls over feet due to unstable balance. He required mod assist x 2 sit ⇆ stand and to maintain static postural control. Mod assist required to complete donning of underwear and coveralls over hips and to place arms in armholes of coveralls while standing. After sitting, resident dependent with zipping and fastening 2 snaps to fasten coveralls 2° fatigue. When performing toileting task, patient required max assist to transfer standing pivot from w/c → toilet. Patient needed max assist x 1 to maintain postural control to doff/don underwear and coveralls to knee level.*

**Write your own "A" and "P" sections for the ADL note below.**

---

**HELPFUL HINT**

Look at every sentence in the "S" and the "O" and decide what each might mean. Note that the therapist used verbal, tactile, and written communication with this patient. What might that tell you? He was too tired to fasten his coveralls after finishing dressing. What does that mean? Also note that he needed max assist to maintain static postural control during parts of the session. What does that mean in terms of his needs and/or his function? His assist levels vary: max assist x 1, max assist x 2, dependent. What is your assessment of that? What treatment do you think would benefit the patient? How often would you want to see him? How long do you think you would want each session to be?

# CHAPTER 9
## Treatment Planning

Now that you know the basics of writing a SOAP note, we will back up a little and give some attention to the treatment planning on which your notes are based. In *Elements of Clinical Documentation* (Revision) (AOTA, 1998a) the treatment or intervention plan is considered one of the three elements of the initial evaluation report. The other two elements are the identification and background information gathering, and the assessment. The treatment plan is described as including the long-term functional goals, short-term goals, the intervention or treatment procedures, the type, amount, frequency, and duration of treatment, as well as recommendations for other services or specialized treatments.

Your critical thinking as an occupational therapist is more evident in the development of the treatment plan than anywhere else in your work. The treatment plan is a creative work in progress. It is a dynamic, creative, joint venture between you and your patient along with the family or significant other when appropriate, and oriented toward the patient's ultimate success in fulfilling his life roles. The treatment plan must be realistic; that is, it must have a good chance of success in a reasonable period of time. It must show evidence of the need for your professional skill. The treatment plan must be discussed with the patient, and together you and the patient must create this plan for achieving the patient's rehabilitation goals and for enabling his occupational performance.

## The Process

From the moment the referral is received, treatment planning begins in the mind of the therapist. A name, age, and reason for referral will stimulate a good occupational therapist to begin reviewing in his mind the areas he is likely to assess, the areas of deficits he might expect to find, and the possible interventions he might want to use. Each individual is different of course, and there will be many variations, as well as some surprises as he begins the assessment. The mental preparation for *"Angus Campbell, age 68, Ⓛ CVA, evaluate and treat"* takes a therapist on a mental journey along one road of thought, whereas *"Lindsey Johnson, age 4, ADHD,"* takes the therapist mentally down a different pathway. From day one, a good therapist also begins discharge planning based on the patient's past life experiences, prior level of functioning, and probable discharge placement.

As soon as the order is received, the therapist documents the referral in the chart and reviews the available information about the patient in preparation for his first visit. The information may be obtained from the chart or a call to the physician or a conversation with the teacher who might have made the referral. It is helpful to know the answers to questions that have already been asked by other professional staff, rather than to ask them again.

The next step is a visit to the patient. In an outpatient setting much information is gleaned from simply watching the patient enter into the treatment area. Does the patient guard for pain? Is a supportive family member accompanying the patient? What is the quality of movement and posture? Are there obvious cognitive or perceptual problems?

If the patient is oriented and verbal, an interview is top on the agenda. If the patient is not able to provide information, the family or other caregiver may be able to provide the information needed. What areas of this patient's life present the most problems? What was the patient able to do prior to this injury or hospitalization? What roles are important to this patient? What does this patient desire from treatment? What results do the family hope to see? What supports are available to make this happen?

From this interview, the therapist begins selecting evaluation tools. First it is important to evaluate function (performance areas) and then underlying factors (performance components). In this way no time will be lost evaluating performance components that do not impact function.

The initial evaluation leads to formulation of a problem list. The therapist and patient agree on the priorities for treatment for this patient at this time. This leads directly to setting goals and choosing treatment interventions. It is also important to know who is paying for your services. Workers' compensation programs are state-supported programs funded by employers to provide for services for a person injured on the job. Therefore, the covered services revolve around treatment focused on the person's ability to return to work. Medicare, on the other hand, is a federally funded insurance program mainly for persons over the age of 65 and provides primarily for the treatment of acute illnesses that result in deficits in self-care. Its recipients are usually retired.

In the public school system where therapy services are mandated by federal laws such as IDEA and where some of the therapy services are funded by Medicaid, occupational therapy treatment may be educationally related treatment that focuses only on the child's functioning in the classroom. Private insurance organizations such as Blue Cross may provide for coverage of services for a wider variety of goals than other payers or may cover occupational therapy only for narrower and more specific treatments for certain diagnoses. All payers, however, are interested in the amount of time that will be needed for treatment and in the cost effectiveness of the treatment.

Documentation of the initial evaluation is provided in whatever format the facility uses. Most practice settings use forms for initial evaluation reports. An example of such a form is found in *Chapter 11: Documention in Different Practice Settings*. The initial evaluation may be handwritten or computerized. It may be a narrative note or a SOAP note. Although initial evaluations are quite lengthy and time-consuming when written in the SOAP format, the information gathered in an initial evaluation fits nicely into the SOAP format.

*S:*     *The interview data*

*O:*     *The evaluation data from both standardized evaluation tools and your clinical observations*

*A:*     *Your professional assessment of the data you reported in "O," your determination of the rehab potential along with the problem list*

From the "S," "O," and "A" the goals and objectives are established, leading to:

*P:*     *Frequency and duration of treatment, along with the intervention strategies for meeting the goals and objectives*

## Estimating Rehab Potential

Rehab potential is always stated as good or excellent for the goals you want to accomplish. If it is not good or excellent for your patient, select a smaller, more incremental goal. There is not much point in setting and working toward goals that you do not have a good chance of accomplishing. Estimating rehab potential as poor, fair, or guarded is a red flag to reviewers and they may be reluctant to set aside health care dollars for someone who is unlikely to benefit. Rehab potential does not mean independence. It means potential to reach the goals you have set or potential for the patient to make significant change.

## Selecting Intervention Strategies

Since selecting strategies and treatment media is a daily task for an occupational therapist, it can seem to an inexperienced therapist almost like reinventing the wheel to select these differently for each individual patient. One of the striking differences between occupational therapy and other disciplines is the way in which strategies and media are selected to meet the patient's goals. In occupational therapy, the task must be meaningful to the individual patient, and selected for its meaningfulness. Occupational therapy is a process of creative problem-solving with each patient in each performance area. What is meaningful to one patient may not be to another.

Even the most basic task such as dressing may not seem meaningful to some patients. A person with tetraplegia who has a personal attendant, for example, may never need to dress himself, and may consider it an enormous waste of time to be required to learn to do so. However, he may be very motivated to learn to hold a cue stick in order to reengage in social activities with his friends. Some patients will never need to balance a checkbook, while others may not be able to return to living independently without this skill. The difference between competent and exceptional occupational therapy may well lie in the ability to find meaningful activities and design these into your treatment strategies.

The occupational therapist asks questions like:

- What do you want to be able to do?
- What keeps you from being able to do that?
- What are the possible options for making that happen?

The options for intervention strategies may include teaching new skills, working to increase performance components (range, strength, and endurance), or modifying the environment. Occupational therapy considers doing things in many different ways. The creativity of the individual therapist comes into play here. How many ways are there to get light into a room if the patient can no longer manage a light switch? How many activities that require wrist extension could be adapted to reach the objective of increasing AROM at the wrist? Would any of these qualify as meaningful to this patient?

The treatment media used by occupational therapy is also different from that used by other disciplines. Occupational therapists often use common household objects to accomplish functional tasks. For example, the patient's own clothing is a common treatment media. The clothes may be used for dressing to teach the patient to don clothing or may be used for folding in order to be doing a meaningful activity while increasing standing tolerance, or for hanging in a closet to increase AROM at the shoulder. The approach would depend upon what the patient will need to do in the setting to which she will be discharged. An experienced occupational therapist can find many different uses for common household objects. The same net ball that is used to wash dishes may be used for squeezing to develop grip strength or for throwing to develop UE range and strength.

## Developing Intervention Strategies

Intervention strategies do not stand alone. Strategies must be based on problems and long-term goals, and they must be purposeful to the patient to be useful. However, for the purpose of learning to generate possible strategies, we will suspend that requirement and think of as many ways as possible to meet a treatment objective. Consider the following:

| STG | Interventions |
|---|---|
| *Pt. will be able to complete basic ADL tasks while standing for 5-minute increments and taking rest breaks as needed by discharge date 3/10/99.* | *1. Set up task to make coffee while standing at counter in the ADL kitchen.*<br>*2. Instruct pt. to stand at the bathroom sink to wash hands after toileting.*<br>*3. Instruct pt. to stand in a standing table to play a game.*<br>*4. Instruct pt. to stand to arrange clothing while dressing in the AM.*<br>*5. Instruct pt. to stand to look out window to watch birds eat the food she has put out.* |
| *Pt. will be able to manage his financial affairs ① in order to live alone after discharge.* | *1. Teach basic math skills (add, subtract, multiply, divide).*<br>*2. Role play to make change correctly.*<br>*3. Set up task for writing checks to pay fabricated bills.*<br>*4. Teach comparison shopping using a catalog.*<br>*5. Set up task of writing out a budget.*<br>*6. Set up task of balancing checkbook.*<br>*7. Set up experience for deciding whether a given amount of money will be enough for living expenses once a set of fabricated bills has been paid.* |

## Contents of the Treatment Plan

The format of the treatment plan will vary from one facility to another. In this manual you will see more than one format for creating a treatment plan. Since the treatment plan is technically a part of the initial evaluation report rather than a document that stands on its own, how much of the demographic and referral data is recorded on the form and how much is recorded elsewhere in the evaluation report varies from one practice setting to another. Somewhere in the evaluation report it is necessary to record the following information.

- Basic demographic data (name, age, sex, date of admission, treatment diagnosis, date of onset of current diagnosis, referring physician)
- Referral source, date of referral, services requested
- Brief history, secondary problems, contraindications, and precautions
- Problems to be addressed (performance area and performance components not WFL)
- Rehab potential (patient's potential to meet the goals you set together)
- Special circumstances which justify occupational therapy
- Person responsible for carrying out or coordinating the treatment
- Expected timelines for reaching goals and objectives
- Prior functional status
- Performance areas to be addressed

On the treatment plan form specifically you will need:

- Long-term functional goals
- Short-term goals
- Interventions or treatment strategies to be used
- Frequency and duration of treatment
- Consumer and family agreement with goals
- Recommendations

## Frequency and Duration of Treatment

Medicare has established "edits" that show the common frequency and duration of treatment by diagnosis. This can be helpful for a new therapist in formulating timelines, even though each individual patient will be different. In working with managed care, a set number of visits will be approved. A therapist must learn to set priorities that will use the approved time to the patient's best advantage. When negotiating for the number of visits to be allowed, it is useful to make a sound case for what you want, backed up by reasons and probable results, and based on the rehab potential. In a long-term care setting where therapy is based on an already established formula of treatment minutes, you will also need to prioritize your treatment goals.

It can sometimes seem impossible to a new therapist to estimate how much time will be needed to accomplish goals. With a little experience you will find that you really can do it. Please remember that the treatment plan is made to be changed. If your original estimate does not turn out to be accurate, you change it as you find out how quickly your patient progresses.

Now you will have an opportunity to look at an example of a treatment plan and practice selecting possible intervention strategies to accomplish the consumer's long- and short-term goals. For purposes of demonstration, the plan used as an example covers only one problem. This would be unusual in a real treatment setting.

# Hospital and Rehabilitation Center Occupational Therapy
# Treatment Plan

**Patient Name:** Marge B.        **Age:** 71        **Sex:** F        **Medical Record #:** 04136
**Primary Diagnosis:** Ⓛ CVA        **Secondary Diagnosis:** Diabetes
**Referring Physician:** F. Dittrich, M.D.        **Date of Treatment Plan:** 1/21/99
**Frequency and Duration of Treatment:** 2 x day for 4 weeks (20 treatment sessions)
**Primary Occupational Therapist:** Charlet Quay, OTR/L
**Problem:** Pt. requires mod Ⓐ in self-care due to inability to spontaneously use Ⓡ UE 2° ⒧CVA.
**Long-Term Goal:** Pt. will be able to complete self-care and IADL activities Ⓘ within 4 weeks.

| STG | Interventions |
|---|---|
| Pt. will demonstrate spontaneous use of Ⓡ UE as a functional assist in self-care within 2 weeks. | 1. Normalize tone through the use of NDT approaches.<br>2. Instruct in sensory stimulation to affected side to ↓ neglect.<br>3. Weight bear on Ⓡ UE while engaged in functional activities that require weight shifts: sorting laundry, playing a board game, turning pages of a magazine.<br>4. Facilitate grasp and release for use of prehension; facilitate reach patterns through handling, joint approximation, guided resistance, and muscle stretch.<br>5. Provide activities that require Ⓡ UE as an assist (stabilizing tablet while writing, stabilizing toothpaste while removing lid) or Ⓑ UE use (wringing out washcloth, applying body lotion). |
| Pt. will dress self with min Ⓐ within 2 weeks using Ⓡ UE as a functional assist. | 1. Instruct in adaptive dressing techniques.<br>2. Instruct in use of Ⓡ UE to stabilize shirt while buttoning, assist in pulling up pants, holding on to bra while hooking in front.<br>3. Instruct in adaptive equipment as needed: long shoe horn, elastic shoe laces, reacher or dressing stick.<br>4. Facilitate trunk control and balance in weight shifts forward and backward, side to side, and in rotational patterns in preparation for and throughout dressing activity as needed. |
| Pt. will be safe in light meal preparation and cleanup with SBA in 3 weeks. | 1. In collaboration with patient and family, adapt kitchen for safe accessibility and mobility.<br>2. Plan meal with attention to money management, organization, and sequencing of component tasks.<br>3. Instruct in functional mobility in kitchen to transport items while preparing lunch using gait patterns learned in PT. Use wheeled cart as needed for efficient and safe transport of items.<br>4. Instruct in correct and safe body mechanics in reaching items in refrigerator, on stovetop, in oven or microwave, and in performing sink, counter top, and cooking activities.<br>5. Instruct in energy conservation during meal preparation and cleanup.<br>6. Select and instruct in use of appropriate adaptive equipment for one-handedness as needed to peel and chop vegetables, open cans and jars. |

| STG | Interventions |
|---|---|
| Pt. will ↑ 2# in Ⓡ tripod pinch strength with pain level of < 5/10 in order to perform work tasks within 2 weeks. | 1.<br><br>2.<br><br>3.<br><br>4.<br><br>5. |
| Pt. will demonstrate an ↑ of 3# in Ⓡ grip strength with a pain level of < 5/10 within 2 weeks in order to grasp items needed for job within 2 weeks. | 1.<br><br>2.<br><br>3.<br><br>4.<br><br>5. |

# Putting it All Together

You have learned each of the elements of treatment planning, from evaluating the client through developing a problem list, setting goals, assessing rehab potential, figuring out what amount of time you will probably need to accomplish the goals, and choosing intervention strategies.

Now it is your turn. Use the following evaluation to develop a treatment plan. First, develop a problem list. Then establish long-term goals and break these down into short-term goals or objectives. Select intervention strategies that seem useful in reaching your goals and decide how often and for how long you will want to see this client. Combine all of these elements into a treatment plan.

# WORKSHEET 9-2

## Treatment Plan for Ginny H.

Use the following evaluation to develop a treatment plan. First, develop a problem list. Then establish long-term goals and break these down into short-term goals or objectives. Select intervention strategies that seem useful in reaching your goals and decide how often and for how long you will want to see this client. Combine all of these elements into a treatment plan.

**Name:** Ginny H.  **Age:** 87  **Sex:** F  **Physician:** B. Garrett, M.D.
**Diagnosis:** Ⓛ subdural hematoma on 4/22/99, hx. of hypertension, hearing loss
**Date of Onset:** 4/22/99  **Date of Referral:** 5/2/99  **Date of Evaluation:** 5/3/99
**Referral Source:** Nursing on 5/2/99
**History:** Prior to her stroke Ginny had been living for the last 10 years with her unmarried daughter, Sue, who is 60 years old, and works full-time. They live in a two-story house with a bathroom on the second floor. Ginny was in acute care and has just been discharged to a rehabilitation program. She expressed a desire to return to her daughter's home. Her daughter has concerns about being able to care for her mother at home. Ginny has Medicare insurance only.

S:  *Pt. expressed frustration when having difficulty brushing teeth. Pt. c/o back pain 2/10 when grooming. Pt.'s daughter said that pt. was Ⓘ in self-care prior to her stroke but has not cooked or done housework for years; further stated pt. has a hearing loss but no hearing aids.*

O:  *Pt. seen in room for initial assessment.*
*Dressing/Grooming: Pt. stood with CGA for 5 min while brushing teeth after setup and 2 verbal cues. Pt. Ⓘ in donning/doffing socks with extra time. Pt. continued to attempt to don Ⓡ sock using the same techniques for several minutes before being successful. Pt. did not attempt an alternative technique. Pt. mod Ⓐ in donning/doffing gown and robe due to difficulty pulling the robe around her back and threading the Ⓡ UE into the sleeve. Pt. required four 30-second rest breaks during dressing activity due to fatigue.*
*Transfers/ambulation: Pt. sit↔stand with SBA and mod Ⓐ for transfer ⇄ bedside commode due to ↓ standing balance when managing clothing. Pt. walked 3 ft. w/c →sink with CGA using walker.*
*UE ROM and Strength: All UE AROM was WNL except for Ⓑ shoulder abduction and flexion which were WFL. Ⓑ UE strength 5/5 overall except 3/5 in shoulder flexion and abduction.*
*Lateral pinch (lb.): Ⓡ 7.5; Ⓛ 9. Tripod pinch (lb.): Ⓡ 4; Ⓛ 7.*
*Grip (lb.): Ⓡ 29; Ⓛ 37.*
*Sensation: Light touch and sharp/dull tests indicated intact sensation Ⓑ. Pt. correctly identified 1/4 objects in the Ⓡ stereognosis test.*
*Coordination: 9 hole peg test: Placing pegs Ⓡ 52; Ⓛ 37. Removal Ⓡ 26; Ⓛ 14*

Write an assessment and plan for this data, as you learned to do in Chapters 7 and 8.

A:

From Borcherding S. *Documentation Manual for Writing SOAP Notes in Occupational Therapy.* © 2000 SLACK Incorporated

P:

**Now complete the treatment plan.**

Frequency and Duration:

Strengths:

Functional Problem Statements:

LTG:

| STGs (Objectives) | Interventions |
| --- | --- |
|  |  |

LTG:

| STGs (Objectives) | Interventions |
| --- | --- |
|  |  |

# Special Cases in Treatment Planning

Some practice settings use treatment plans that are specific to the population being served. Three of these (mental health, school-based practice, and long-term care) will be discussed in Chapter 11, and examples of the kinds of treatment plans used in these settings will be presented there. Another specialized kind of treatment plan that is becoming increasingly popular as time becomes more precious is the critical care pathway.

# The Critical Care Pathway

In response to the changing health care payment systems, many facilities have developed a form of a standardized treatment plan called a "critical care pathway." Certain kinds of illnesses, surgeries, and disabilities follow a predictable course of recovery. The body responds in a similar way to the condition, even though each person's experience will be unique. Critical care pathways are part of overall quality improvement efforts in health care facilities. In striving for quality care in the most cost-effective manner, the focus of health care is on the outcomes of that care and on the major components that are involved in the delivery of the care (AOTA Managed Care Project Team, 1996).

The goals of critical care pathways and the other monitoring involved in quality improvement programs are to provide some predictability in outcomes, to establish a system of integrating care provided by a myriad of disciplines, and to allow for comparative analysis of treatment and treatment settings. The format of the pathways allows for monitoring a patients' progress on a comparative basis (AOTA Managed Care Project Team, 1996).

In addition to standardizing treatment and establishing checkpoints along a timeline, the use of a standard treatment plan also is more efficient by avoiding unnecessary time spent in rewriting basically the same treatment plan for routine treatment approaches. The standardized plan does allow for adaptations to accommodate individual patient differences, such as multiple diagnoses.

Critical care pathways are usually established to be multidisciplinary but may be specific to occupational therapy. In a setting like a skilled nursing facility that primarily has patients with Medicare insurance coverage, the treatment and patient education provided by each discipline is usually designed to be completed in an allotted number of days that are established by the Diagnostic Related Grouping (DRG) system. An orthopedic unit in an acute care hospital may establish the number of days of treatment based on a retrospective analysis of the hospital's medical records of orthopedic hospitalizations.

## Critical Care Pathways in Rehabilitation

Some diagnoses, such as CVA, are too complex to use a standardized approach to treatment. Other diagnoses, such as a total hip replacement, are very compatible with the critical care pathway system. A critical care pathway for a patient with a total hip replacement resembles the example in Table 9-1.

---

# Table 9-1
## Critical Care Pathway—Total Hip Replacement

**Day One (admission to rehab, post surgery)**
- Initial evaluation
- Film on total hip precautions
- Review precautions and have patient demonstrate to insure understanding

**Day Two**
- Skilled instruction in functional mobility while following hip precautions
- Assess, provide, and instruct in necessary adaptive equipment
- Begin upper extremity strengthening
- Begin ADL training (dressing, grooming, hygiene)

**Day Three**
- Continue UE strengthening
- Continue ADL training
- Skilled instruction in tub and shower transfers
- Introduce home program and have patient demonstrate to insure understanding

**Day Four**
- Skilled instruction in car transfers and stair climbing
- Home evaluation for safety
- Reassess patient's understanding of home program

**Day Five**
- Discharge

---

# Common Errors in Writing Treatment Plans

## Problem Identification
- Problems identified in the assessment are not addressed in the plan.
- Problems are not stated in terms of behavioral manifestations, performance areas, and performance components.
- The number of visits or units requested does not match the severity of the problems.

## Goals
- Goals that are not functional or do not focus on the reason for admission to occupational therapy.
- Treatment plan that does not focus on specific rehabilitation goals that will increase a client's ability to function in the probable discharge environment.
- Goals that focus on the client participating in or cooperating with treatment (unless the client is in the habit of refusing treatment).
- Goals that cannot be measured or do not have a target date for completion.

## Treatment Interventions
- Interventions that do not focus on increasing functional behaviors in order to return the client to the least restrictive environment.
- Interventions that do not take into account the age, sex, and interests of the client or that are not meaningful to the client.
- Acquisition of skills that are not transferred into more functional areas of a client's life.

## Client Involvement

- Noninvolvement of the client in the treatment planning process. The client's signature on the treatment plan indicating that client has read it is not enough to indicate significant client involvement.
- Treatment plan does not reflect the client's strengths, desires, and preferences.

## Canned Plans

- Canned treatment plans that reflect the same goals, objectives, and interventions for each client based on the services available rather than on client need. Even critical pathways need to be individualized to fit the client.

# CHAPTER 10
## Documenting Different Stages of Treatment

As we discussed in *Chapter 2: Documenting the Treatment Process in Occupational Therapy*, different stages of the treatment process require occupational therapists to write different kinds of notes. Very early in the process, an **intake note** may be written acknowledging the referral and stating a plan to evaluate. Next, an **initial evaluation report** is written, reporting the findings from the therapist's evaluation of the patient and detailing a problem list. From this comes the **treatment plan**, which is developed and technically a part of the initial evaluation report. Facilities vary in the type and frequency of **progress notes** required. Some settings, such as home health and outpatient clinics, require a **treatment note** for each visit. Others, such as a mental health, require **progress notes** at least weekly, and more often if changes in status indicate. Long-term care residential facilities usually require a progress note every 30 days, and more frequently for new referrals. The requirements for type and frequency of notes are usually a function of the accrediting agency and the payment source. Sometimes a **reassessment note** is required at regular intervals. Most facilities require a **discharge report** at the end of treatment.

In actual practice, you will find that treatment, progress, and reassessment notes may have some overlap. For example, in outpatient settings the treatment notes often include the client's progress. Treatment notes in other settings where patients may change quickly, such as acute care, may also read much like progress notes. In some ways, progress notes reassess the patient and may sound much like reassessment notes. There are some guidelines for each kind of note, however, and in this chapter we will examine the requirements for documentation at each stage of patient care.

In *Elements of Clinical Documentation* (Revision) (AOTA, 1998a) criteria for five kinds of notes are described—the initial evaluation report (including the treatment plan), treatment notes (also called visit or contact notes), progress reports, reevaluation reports, and discharge or discontinuation reports. In the following exercises we will compare some notes to the AOTA criteria that has been set for them, and see how well the notes stand up under scrutiny.

## Initial Evaluation Reports

After a referral form is received on a patient, you begin the evaluation process of finding out what that patient needs from occupational therapy. First, you collect data from the patient, the family, the chart, and any other pertinent sources. Then you select and administer any standardized tests or survey instruments that will help you determine exactly what needs to be done. From your initial evaluation reports, you identify and prioritize the performance areas and performance components to be treated, and develop a treatment plan. The three elements making up the initial evaluation report as listed in the *Elements of Clinical Documentation* (Revision) (AOTA, 1998a) are as follows:

1. The identifying data and background information
2. The tests performed and clinical observations, followed by your assessment of the results
3. The treatment plan

Most facilities provide a form for an initial evaluation report, and you record your evaluation results on the form, along with comments and observations. Some facilities use the same form for discharge notes so that the evaluation material does not have to be rewritten. The evaluation discharge form from Capital Region Medical Center in Jefferson City, MO is included so you can see what might be included on a good facility form (Figure 10-1a and b). You will notice that it has the performance area evaluations first, followed by performance components, with room for individualization.

**CAPITAL REGION MEDICAL CENTER**
**OCCUPATIONAL THERAPY**
☐ **INITIAL EVALUATION** ☐ **DISCHARGE SUMMARY**

DIAGNOSIS _____ ONSET: _____

MED. HX: _____

_____ CODE STATUS: _____

RELEVANT SURG. PROC.: _____

REFERRAL DATE: _____ DATE: _____

REFERRING PHYSICIAN: _____ MEDICARE #: _____

**ACTIVITIES OF DAILY LIVING**                     REHAB POTENTIAL: _____

| DRESSING<br>Put on & remove the following | INDEP | SBA | MIN. ASSIST | MOD. ASSIST | MAX. ASSIST | ADAPT. EQUIP. | COMMENTS/ADAPTIVE EQUIPMENT ISSUED |
|---|---|---|---|---|---|---|---|
| front opening shirt | | | | | | | |
| pull on shirt | | | | | | | |
| underwear | | | | | | | |
| bra | | | | | | | |
| pants/slacks | | | | | | | |
| socks/hose | | | | | | | |
| shoes | | | | | | | |
| manage fasteners | | | | | | | |
| braces/splints/prosthesis | | | | | | | |
| **GROOMING/HYGIENE** | | | | | | | |
| sponge bath | | | | | | | |
| tub/shower bath | | | | | | | |
| shave | | | | | | | |
| comb hair | | | | | | | |
| brushing teeth | | | | | | | |
| opens jars/bottles | | | | | | | |
| make-up | | | | | | | |
| **EATING** | | | | | | | |
| drink from cup/glass | | | | | | | |
| feeds self | | | | | | | |
| cuts meat | | | | | | | |

**UPPER EXTREMITY ROM & STRENGTH**

| ROM ACTIVE LEFT | PASSIVE LEFT | ACTIVE RIGHT | PASSIVE RIGHT | | | STRENGTH L | R |
|---|---|---|---|---|---|---|---|
| | | | | SHOULDER: | Elevation | | |
| | | | | | Flexion | | |
| | | | | | Abduction | | |
| | | | | | Horizontal Abduction | | |
| | | | | | Horizontal Adduction | | |
| | | | | | Internal Rotation | | |
| | | | | | External Rotation | | |
| | | | | ELBOW: | Flexion | | |
| | | | | | Extension | | |
| | | | | | Supination | | |
| | | | | | Pronation | | |
| | | | | WRIST: | Flexion | | |
| | | | | Shoulder Subluxation | L | R | |
| | | | | UE Edema | L | R | |
| | | | | Pain | L | R | |

**PERTINENT FINDINGS**

Wears glasses _____ Dentures _____ Hearing _____

**MUSCLE TONE/UPPER EXTREMITIES**

Hypotonic _____ Normal _____ Hypertonic _____
Comments _____

**UPPER EXTREMITY SENSATION**

| SENSATION | Intact | Impaired | Absent |
|---|---|---|---|
| Light touch | | | |
| Sharp/Dull | | | |
| Temperature | | | |
| Proprioception | | | |
| Stereognosis | | | |

**COORDINATION/UPPER EXTREMITIES**

Tremors _____ Apraxia _____ Ataxic _____

| | Impaired | WNL |
|---|---|---|
| Gross Motor | | |
| Fine Motor | | |
| 9 Hole Peg Test | L | R |
| Grip Strength | L | R |
| Lateral Pinch | L | R |
| Tripod Pinch | L | R |
| Hand Dominance | L | R |

**ORIENTED TO:**

Person _____ Place _____
Time: Month _____ Day _____ Year _____
Situation _____

**COMMUNICATION/COGNITION**

| | YES | NO |
|---|---|---|
| Verbal | | |
| Understandable | | |
| Appropriate | | |
| Perseveration | | |
| Follows Simple Commands | | |
| Reads | | |
| Writes | | |

2,605.003 (9/99) INIT. EVAL/DISCHG. SUM. (FRONT)

**PERCEPTION**

A. R/L Neglect _____

| | Impaired | WNL |
|---|---|---|
| B. Body Schema | | |
| C. Discrimination | | |
| Shape | | |
| Size | | |
| Color | | |
| D. Visual Perception | | |

Overall Endurance    WFL _____
                     Fair _____
                     Poor _____

| SURVIVAL SKILLS | Indep. | Min. Assist | Mod. Assist | Max. Assist |
|---|---|---|---|---|
| Phone Book Usage | | | | |
| Money Mngmt. | | | | |
| Situational Problem Solving | | | | |
| Homemaking | | | | |

Figure 10-1a. Occupational therapy initial evaluation and discharge summary form (page 1). Courtesy of Capital Region Medical Center, Jefferson City, MO.

HOME SITUATION:_____

LIVING ARRANGEMENTS: (PT ADDRESS) _____

HOME TYPE:_____

PRIOR FUNCTIONAL INDEP.: _____

_____

_____

LEISURE INTERESTS: _____

ADAPTIVE EQUIP.:_____

COMMENTS:_____

_____

_____

_____

PATIENT / FAMILY GOALS:_____

❏ INITIAL ASSESSMENT (PROBLEMS / STRENGTHS)    ❏ DISCHARGE STATUS OF SHORT / LONG TERM GOALS

_____

_____

_____

_____

_____

PLAN:_____

SHORT-TERM GOALS - ESTIMATED TIME TO ACHIEVE: _____

_____

_____

_____

_____

_____

❏ LONG-TERM GOALS - ESTIMATED TIME TO ACHIEVE:    ❏ RECOMMENDATIONS:

_____

_____

_____

_____

_____

❏ Yes    ❏ No    Patient has participated in evaluation process and agrees with treatment plan as stated above.

Therapist _____ Date_____

I have reviewed and agree with the treatment plan as stated above.

Physician Signature _____ Date_____

2,605,003  (9/99)  OT INITIAL EVALUATION/DISCHARGE SUMMARY (BACK)

Figure 10-1b. Occupational therapy initial evaluation and discharge summary form (page 2). Courtesy of Capital Region Medical Center, Jefferson City, MO.

If you are writing an initial evaluation as a SOAP note, this is the way you would categorize your information.

S: **The interview material**
Depending upon your patient's cognitive abilities, you might ask about functioning in all performance areas (ADL, work, and leisure), to determine which are important to the patient and payer, and which are (or are not) WFL in the opinion of your patient. Your interview will also tell you how the patient feels about the problem areas. There may be symbolic losses to consider, as well as physical losses. Perhaps the injury or illness diminishes the patient's view of his own ability to carry out an important role (professional, mate, etc.). You will want to be sensitive to emotional components in the interview. If the patient feels that his injury makes him "less of a man," for example, this could be an important factor in treatment. If you are evaluating a young child or a patient whose cognitive function is not adequate to provide this information, you would need to supplement with information provided by the primary caregivers.

O: **The test results and clinical observations**
This section includes the results of any survey instruments or standardized tests you have performed (such as an ADL evaluation, developmental testing, goniometric evaluation, etc.) along with your clinical observations. Which tests you select will depend entirely on the kind of patient, presenting problem, and situation you are seeing. You would use a very different evaluation battery in long-term care, for example, than you would in the public schools or in a mental health center. Your clinical observations supplement your test results. Quality of movement, for example, may be a very important factor, but not very testable. Your patient may be mod Ⓐ in dressing, but it is important to know that the mod Ⓐ is for balance rather than for motor planning deficits, since those will require very different kinds of treatment.

A: **Your professional assessment of the data presented in the "S" and the "O"**
In this section of your note, you will present your interpretation of the impact of your "O" data on the patient's occupational performance. You will note the performance areas and the performance components that are not WFL. You will note the type and severity of the limitations and the occupational performance deficits caused by these impairments, and set priorities. You will note the rehab potential and justify the need for skilled OT.

Some facilities ask for a problem list in this section of the note. In a facility that uses a POMR, the problem list will be a separate document. In some settings (such as mental health centers and public school) the problem list is multidisciplinary. The problem list must be included somewhere in your records, as it will be the basis for formulating a treatment plan, with each problem being expanded to include long and short-term goals and interventions to address the stated problem. Some facilities put the long and short-term goals in the "A" section of the note, although most put them under the "P."

P: **Frequency and duration of planned treatment and the long- and short-term goals**
If you have not already noted your long- and short-term goals for the patient, you will do this under the "P." You will set priorities. Safety, for example, is often a top priority. Reduction of pain is often another high priority item. Some kinds of performance components are prerequisites for the development of other. For example, sitting balance is a prerequisite for any task that must be done while sitting. Function is critical to the plan. As OTs we are reimbursed for increasing occupational performance, and this must be reflected in the plan.

Discharge planning also begins with the initial evaluation. From the inception of care, you will plan toward the probable discharge situation. This may change over the course of the patient's time in occupational therapy, but it is always a consideration.

The problems and goals noted in the "A" and "P" sections of your note form the foundation of your treatment plan. The treatment plan will change as the patient progresses, but as soon as you have completed your initial evaluation, you have an idea of which areas of deficit you plan to address, along with the goals you and the patient have agreed are most important at the present time.

The *Elements of Clinical Documentation* (Revision) (AOTA, 1998a) states that an initial evaluation should contain basic demographic data, both the current diagnosis and the treatment diagnosis, the date of onset, the date and source of referral, along with the services that are being requested. Some physicians are very specific in requesting service, e.g., "fabricate resting cockup splint," while others may simply say "evaluate and treat." The initial evaluation should contain a history along with any precautions or contraindications. In most practice settings, much of the demographic and referral data is contained elsewhere in the medical record and is not repeated on the initial evaluation report form. Some facilities use an addressograph card that stamps the demographic data onto each sheet of the medical record. Other facilities have a place for it on one of the forms used. If you are in private practice, you will need to make certain that all the required data is present in some part of your evaluation report.

You will notice that several formats for initial evaluation reports are used in this manual. There are many correct ways to format the information, and different facilities may choose to organize the information in any manner they like as long as it is all present. The different formats are provided to make it clear that there is no one "correct" organizational strategy.

Examination by the therapist should include the current level of function in all performance areas and contexts tested, as well as a statement about what the consumer and his family expect from treatment. The results of all tests should be noted along with any other sources of information. For example, the patient and family might have provided information in an interview. In a SOAP note, this would be your "S" and "O" data. Then the test results and information gathered should be interpreted. You will list the type and severity of the impairments and the functional limitations these cause. This would be the "A" section of your SOAP note. Next you will determine rehab potential. Remember that the rehab potential is not the potential to be independent, but rather the potential to reach the goals you and the patient set. If rehab potential is not good, you should reevaluate your goals.

From this information, you will make a treatment plan containing the long- and short-term goals, the interventions you plan to use, the frequency and duration of treatment, and any recommendations you have.

Under the current Prospective Payment System (PPS) used by Medicare in long-term care settings, the time spent in initial evaluation is becoming shorter in order to allow for treatment to begin sooner, and this is beginning to impact the amount of data that is initially collected. Our challenge as we move into the 21st century is to be as complete as we can in evaluating a client in the amount of time we have to get it done.

Read the following initial evaluation report and treatment plan. Use the checklist in Worksheet 10-1 to evaluate the report against the criteria described in the *Elements of Clinical Documentation* (Revision) (AOTA, 1998a).

# Hospital and Rehabilitation Center Occupational Therapy Initial Evaluation Report

**Name:** Agnes H.  **Age:** 68  **Sex:** F  **Physician:** T. Quay, M.D.
**Date of Onset:** 2/1/98 **Date of Admission:** 2/2/98 **Date of Evaluation:** 2/3/98 **Time:** 10 am
**History:** Pt. referred by Dr. Quay for evaluation and treatment. She was admitted after a fall resulting in confusion and left-sided weakness. Prior to admission she was living alone and was Ⓘ in all activities of daily living.
**Primary Diagnosis:** Ⓡ CVA r/o OBS  **Secondary Diagnosis:** diabetes

**S:** Pt. stated, "I'm doing this so I can go home."

**O:** Pt. seen at bedside for mini mental status exam, manual muscle test, AROM, strength, and functional mobility. Pt. also seen in shower room for toileting, dressing ⇆ undressing and showering.
**Bathing:** Upper body: min Ⓐ  Lower body: min Ⓐ  except max Ⓐ for perineal area and feet.
**Dressing:** Seated in chair with arms, min Ⓐ with verbal cues except for mod Ⓐ to initiate donning bra, and max Ⓐ for shoes and socks. Verbal cues needed for sequencing and environment orientation.
**Toileting:** Verbal cues to flush, min Ⓐ to obtain tissue and manage clothing.
**Transfers:** CGA with verbal cues for safety/proper arm placement sit to stand; min Ⓐ from low surfaces.
**Bed Mobility:** Rolls & supine ⇆ sit SBA
**Standing Balance:** static: CGA
**Activity Tolerance:** fair (3) (1-5 scale) 10 minutes max tolerance to any activity with physical/mental challenges.
**Motor Planning/Perception:** WFLs
**Cognition:** Score of 17/30 on MME. Sequencing problems during dressing tasks noted. Pt. could not attach bra in back and required verbal cues to attach in front.
**UE AROM:** WFLs for all Ⓑ UE movements except: abd, int/ext. rotation of Ⓛ shoulder.
**UE Strength:** Grip: Ⓡ 42 lbs. Ⓛ 21 lbs. Pinch: Ⓡ palmar 14#; Ⓡ lateral 15#; Ⓛ palmar 6 #; Ⓛ lateral 8#
**Manual Muscle Test:** All movements 4/5 except Ⓛ elbow ext. 3/5, thumb opposition and abduction 3+
**Sensation:** Ⓛ UE: Light touch, pain, temperature intact; Stereognosis 3/5 Ⓡ UE all intact

**A:** Pt. problem-solved poorly while undressing, (trying to doff pants prior to doffing shoes/socks) and during dressing to initiate an alternative way to don bra. Pt. displayed Ⓛ UE ↓ AROM, ↓ strength, slow cognition and sequencing and problem-solving strategies. Pt. has ↓ short-term memory, which is a safety concern. Due to ↓ cognition pt. requires verbal cues to initiate some ADL tasks. Pt. would benefit from environmental cues to orient her to environment, problem-solving, and sequencing activities, and activities to ↑ AROM and strength in the Ⓛ UE. Rehab potential is good for modified Ⓘ in ADL activities.

**P:** Pt. will be seen for 45 minute sessions 5 x wk. for 2 wks. for sequencing during ADL tasks, problem-solving strategies, activities to ↑ activity tolerance, AROM and strength in Ⓛ UE. Put calender in pt.'s room to increase orientation to month, day, and season. Pt. will be able to dress with SBA and < 3 verbal cues after set up within 2 weeks.

Tara Grantham, OTR/L

# Treatment Plan

**Problem #1:** Pt. needs min to max physical assist and verbal cues to dress self due to ↓ AROM, activity tolerance, and ability to sequence the task.
**Long-Term Goal:** Pt. will be able to dress with SBA and < 3 verbal cues after set up within 2 weeks.

| STG (Objective) | Interventions |
|---|---|
| Pt. will don bra ① using adapted technique within 1 week. | 1. Teach adaptive techniques.<br>2. Post picture of how to don bra correctly using adapted technique.<br>3. Reinforce correct responses.<br>4. Teach coordination exercises. |
| Pt. will don shoes and socks ① using adapted technique and a long shoehorn within 1½ weeks. | 1. Provide long shoehorn and instruct pt. in correct use.<br>2. Instruct in adapted techniques for donning shoes and socks.<br>3. Post picture of adapted technique and long shoehorn being used to don shoes.<br>4. Instruct in using affected side as a functional assist in dressing.<br>5. Expand exercise program to include AROM and strength. |
| Pt. will sequence dressing tasks correctly 3/3 tries within 2 weeks. | 1. Verbalize steps before beginning to dress.<br>2. Verbalize steps while dressing.<br>3. Post list of steps for pt. to follow.<br>4. Take rest breaks as needed for activity tolerance. |

**Problem #2:** Pt.'s lack of orientation to environment and inability to problem-solve cause safety concerns with ADL and home management.
**Long-Term Goal:** Pt. will correctly use calendar, schedule, clock, and emergency information posted on wall within 2 weeks.

| STG (Objective) | Interventions |
|---|---|
| Pt. will correctly identify time, date, and situation when asked within 1 week. | 1. Post calendar, schedule, and emergency information near clock in pt.'s room.<br>2. Instruct nursing staff and other therapy staff to ask pt. date, time, and situation several times daily and to reinforce correct responses. |
| Pt. will be able to follow a daily schedule with < 2 verbal cues within 1½ weeks. | 1. Post daily schedule on wall near clock.<br>2. Cue pt. to look at schedule to determine what she should be doing at any given time. |
| Pt. will correctly problem-solve responses to emergency situations with 90% accuracy within 2 weeks. | 1. Provide situations for patient to problem-solve, progressing from easy to more complex.<br>2. Provide telephone directory or other props as needed for problem-solving. |

# WORKSHEET 10-1

## Initial Evaluation Report

**In each section on the right side of the checklist, make a note of the item in the evaluation that meets the criteria.**

### Background Data

| Criteria | Compliance |
|---|---|
| Is the basic demographic data (name, age, sex, date of onset, date of admission, date of referral) present? Note any not present.<br><br>Who referred the patient to OT, on what date, and what services were requested?<br><br>Is the patient's history and prior level of function included?<br><br>Are there any secondary problems, pre-existing conditions, contraindications, or precautions that will impact therapy?<br><br>What life stage or environmental factors will impact treatment?<br><br>Is the current level of function assessed?<br><br>What do the consumer and her family expect or want from treatment? | |

Adapted from *Elements of Clinical Documentation* (Revision) (AOTA, 1998a)

### Results of the Assessment

| Criteria | Compliance |
|---|---|
| What tests were used? Were there any deviations from the standard procedures?<br><br>Was any other information collected besides that from the tests?<br><br>Are the impairments and their severity identified?<br><br>Are the functional limitations stated in objective and measurable terms?<br><br>Is the rehab potential noted? | |

Adapted from *Elements of Clinical Documentation* (Revision) (AOTA, 1998a)

*Treatment Plan*

| Criteria | Compliance |
|---|---|
| How well do the long-term goals meet the standards you have been taught? | |
| Are the long-term goals reasonable in relation to the consumer's current status, rehabilitation status, and prior level of functioning? | |
| What documentation is there that the patient and family agree with the goals? | |
| Do the short-term goals (objectives) relate to the long-term goals? | |
| How well do the objectives meet the standards you have been taught? | |
| Are the interventions that have been selected appropriate to meet the goals? | |
| What assistive devices are to be used? | |
| What is the number, frequency, and duration of treatment? | |
| Are there any recommendations or referrals? | |

Adapted from *Elements of Clinical Documentation* (Revision) (AOTA, 1998a)

## Treatment Notes

Contact, visit, or treatment notes are used to document each visit or each individual occupational therapy session. In some situations, such as home health, contact notes are required in the medical record each time a patient is seen. In other cases, such as mental health, the occupational therapist keeps attendance records and informal contact notes, which he uses for the purpose of summarizing them into a progress note.

Contact notes should contain documentation of the attendance and participation of the consumer in therapy. If the consumer did not attend as scheduled, there should be a note of the reason therapy did not occur. The interventions used in therapy should be noted, along with the consumer's response. If any assistive or adaptive devices were used, these should be noted, along with their effectiveness. It is possible that some items will not apply in all situations. For example, in a mental health setting there may not be any assistive or adaptive equipment used.

Read the following treatment note and use Worksheet 10-2 to determine how well it meets the standards.

# Hospital and Rehabilitation Center Acute Care Unit
# Occupational Therapy Contact Note

**Date:** 4/14/99          **Time:** 8:30 AM

**S:** Pt. reports, "I feel fair today. I had a long night."

**O:** Pt. seen bedside in ICU for instruction in ADL tasks and AROM in Ⓡ UE. Pt. nodded his head when asked if ready to sit up; required mod Ⓐ supine → sit. Upon sitting $O_2$ saturation dropped to ~ 85%. Grooming, dressing, and UE AROM activities not completed 2° low $O_2$ levels. Pt. given min Ⓐ to return to supine. After ~2 minutes $O_2$ levels returned to ~95%. Pt. washed face p̄ set up in supine and nodded when asked if that felt good.

**A:** Pt. able to tolerate a little more activity today than yesterday when he did not have tolerance for supine → sit. Pt. also appears more motivated to attempt therapy session. Activity tolerance still limited due to $O_2$ saturation levels upon exertion. Pt. would benefit from instruction in energy conservation as well as correct positioning to ↓ exertion ↑ activity tolerance for ADL tasks.

**P:** Continue skilled OT qd to ↑ activity tolerance, and Ⓘ in ADL tasks for 5 days or until d/c. Pt. will complete grooming EOB c̄ rest breaks as needed within 2 treatment sessions.

Bonnie Student, OTR/L

# WORKSHEET 10-2

## Contact, Visit, or Treatment Notes

Using the following checklist, determine whether or not the note on page 109 meets the standards for treatment notes.

| Criteria | Compliance |
|---|---|
| What evidence is there of the patient's participation in OT treatment? | |
| What activities, techniques, or modalities were used in this treatment session? | |
| If any assistive or adaptive devices were used, is there documentation of whether these were fabricated, sold, or rented, their effectiveness, and what the instructions were for its use? | |
| How did this patient (consumer) respond to the treatment provided? | |

Adapted from *Elements of Clinical Documentation* (Revision) (AOTA, 1998a)

# Progress Notes

Progress notes are written on a regularly scheduled basis, (usually weekly or monthly) with the time frame determined by the facility. The facility is guided by the accrediting agencies and primary payers in setting the time frame in which progress notes must be written. The requirements for a progress note require that the treatment interventions be specified, along with the consumer's response to them. There should be an explanation of goals that are modified or changed or continued, along with any changes in expected time frames. The effectiveness of treatment including any adaptive devices should be noted. Any conferences with others should be documented, any home programs should be attached, and any instruction given to caregivers should be noted, along with future plans (AOTA, 1998a).

# Behavioral Health Center Occupational Therapy Progress Note

**S:**     *In assertion group on Tuesday 10/11/99, pt. talked about how her life had taken a "downward spiral" since early September, and she had become more passive and less proactive in getting her needs met, although she had not been aware of it at the time.*

**O:**     *Pt. attended assertion group 2/2, communication group 1/1, and ADL group 3/5 this week. She was on time to 4/6 groups without reminders, wearing neatly pressed clothing, makeup, and an ornament in her hair. In assertion group on Thursday 10/12 she shared (without prompting) 2 stories about her usual way of dealing with retail situations. In communication group she spontaneously answered one question addressed to the group as a whole, and in ADL group she offered to assist another pt. with his checkbook.*

**A:**     *Pt.'s spontaneous actions in groups and willingness to share verbally seem to indicate an improved mood this week. Her unprompted attendance is up this week from 2/8 to 6/8 groups. Her improved dress, hygiene, and makeup also indicate an improvement in mood from last week. Pt. would benefit from planning a structure for her days to prevent another "downward spiral" after discharge.*
*Goals #1 (assertion) and #2 (communication) are met as of this date.*
*Goal #3 (leisure skills) is continued through discharge on 10/19/99 pending formulation of a plan.*
*Goal #4 (ADL) was discontinued on 10/11/99.*

**P:**     *Pt. to be seen in groups for 3 more days, with discharge anticipated on Wednesday of next week. ADL group will be used for preparing the structured plan for using her time. Pt. will prepare a plan including at least one planned activity per day for at least 5 days out of 7 after discharge and will discuss it with her husband and social worker by discharge on 10/19/99.*

Sharon Young, COTA

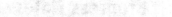

# WORKSHEET 10-3

## *Progress Notes*

Using the following checklist, determine whether or not the note on page 113 meets the standards for progress notes.

| Criteria | Compliance |
|---|---|
| What treatment interventions were used? | |
| What change has occurred in this consumer? | |
| What goals have been continued, what goals have been changed, and what goals have been discontinued? | |
| Have there been any changes in the time frames for reaching goals? | |
| If any assistive devices are being used, how effective are these? | |
| What contact or conferences have there been with others? | |
| Is there is a home program, or instructions given to caregivers? | |
| If there is a home program, is it attached, and is there documentation of the consumer's ability to follow it? | |
| Is there a specific plan for the future? | |

Adapted from *Elements of Clinical Documentation* (Revision) (AOTA, 1998a)

## Reevaluation Reports

In some settings, patients must be reevaluated monthly or quarterly. The reassessment report is a cross between a progress note and a discharge summary. The tests that were given initially are readministered and the results are compared with the results of the previous tests to determine the effectiveness of the treatment being provided. The goals and plans are revised at this time and new time lines are projected.

Read the reevaluation report that follows and use Worksheet 10-4 to determine how well it meets the AOTA criteria. In addition, see whether this note meets the other standards for a good OT note that you have been taught in the previous chapters of this manual.

# Hospital and Rehabilitation Center Reassessment Report

S: *Pt. initially reported "numbness and tingling in fingers." During last tx. session pt. reported his " Ⓛ hand feels much stronger now."*

O: *Pt. admitted to hospital on 1/26/98 for treatment of Ⓛ UE following closed head injury resulting from MVA. OT initial evaluation on 1/27/98. Reassessment on 2/5/98. ADL assessment attached.*

|  | Ⓛ UE:  1/26 | Ⓡ UE: WNL  2/5 |
|---|---|---|
| Shoulder Flexion | F | F+ |
| Shoulder Extension | F | G |
| Shoulder Abd | F | F+ |
| Shoulder Add | F | N |
| Internal Rotation | F+ | G |
| External Rotation | F+ | G |
| Horizontal Abd | F | G |
| Horizontal Add | F | G |
| Elbow Flexion | F- | F+ |
| Elbow Extension | F- | F+ |
| Pronation | F- | F + |
| Supination | F- | G- |
| Wrist Flexion | F- | G- |
| Wrist Extension | F | G |
| L Grip | 30/30/25 | 40/40/35 |
| L Lateral Pinch | 8/8/7 | 10/11/10 |
| L Palmar Pinch | 6.5/6.5/7.5 | 8/7/8 |

*Pt. has been seen b.i.d. to work on strengthening the Ⓛ UE using Thera-Band, hand held wt. exercises, and putty to increase independence in both basic and instrumental ADLs. Pt. has also worked on improving standing balance and has been instructed in bathroom safety (as related to tub transfers and equipment needs), but has not yet demonstrated proficiency in this area due to ↓ balance and activity tolerance.*

A:     Pt. (L) muscle strength, grip strength, and prehension patterns have all improved. Pt. now able to continue exercise program under supervision of rehab aide.
Goals #1 and #2 are met.
Goal #3 (balance) not yet met.
Goal #4 (min (A) in ADLs) changed to (I) in ADLs.
Pt. shows excellent rehab potential to return home to live with spouse safely after one more week of treatment. Pt. would benefit from continued work on balance and activity tolerance, long handled sponge and bath bench and instruction in use, as well as home eval and design home exercise program.

P:     One additional week of b.i.d. treatment is requested in order to work on ↑ balance and activity tolerance needed for (I) in ADLs, and to complete home eval, design home exercise program.

Tammie Student, OTR/L

# WORKSHEET 10-4

## Reevaluation Report

Using the following checklist, determine whether or not the note on pages 117 and 118 meets the standards for reevaluation reports.

| Criteria | Compliance |
|---|---|
| What tests were readministered and what were the results? | |
| How do the current findings compare to the previous results? | |
| What are the changes in anticipated functional outcomes? | |
| What revisions are being made in the goals, objectives, and interventions? | |
| What revisions are being made in the frequency and duration of treatment? | |

Adapted from *Elements of Clinical Documentation* (Revision) (AOTA, 1998a)

## Discharge Summaries

A discharge summary (also called a discontinuation report) is used to summarize the course of a patient's treatment and to make recommendations for referral or follow-up care. Discharge notes often follow a format of their own, stating why and when the patient was referred, giving a summary of the initial findings, the course of treatment followed by a summary of progress, and any recommendations for follow-up care.

Given the time constraints and productivity standards common in practice today, you might wonder why writing a note on a patient who is no longer on the caseload would be considered a good use of your time. Typically there are several reasons. First, the patient may be discharged to a less restrictive level of care rather than to home, and from one OT to another while still requiring treatment. For example, an OT providing acute care might discharge a patient to the OT who is providing rehab care. The OT doing rehab care then discharges the patient to the OT providing home health care. Ideally, each OT is able to use the discharge summary to build on skills developed under the previous therapist's care.

Even if the patient is discharged home or to a situation that does not include further OT services, the patient may need to be readmitted at a later time. If you receive a referral on a readmitted patient who was not previously on your caseload, it is very helpful to know what was done, what gains were made, and how the patient responded, along with what worked and what did not. In some cases, the doctor who made the referral may be the only follow-up available for the patient. In addition to providing follow-up care to his patient, he may want to know how his referral for OT was handled, what benefit has accrued to his patient, and whether to use OT in the future.

According to *Elements of Clinical Documentation* (Revision) (AOTA, 1998a), discharge summaries should contain a summary of the course of treatment, including the number of treatment sessions and the consumer's response. The goals and objectives are examined to see whether they were achieved, fully or partially. Current functional status is compared to functional status prior to therapy. Any home programs and follow-up plans are noted, and recommendations and referrals are made.

Discharge summaries may be done as SOAP notes, or the facility may have a particular form or format that is to be used. We will be evaluating one that is in a SOAP format and a one that is done on a facility form. Some facilities use the same form for admission and discharge, making it quicker to prepare the discharge report.

Read the following discharge summaries and use Worksheets 10-5 and 10-6 to determine whether these summaries meet the AOTA criteria.

# Hospital and Rehabilitation Center Discharge Summary

**Date:** 2/19/99          **Time:** 9:00 AM

**S:**   Pt. said, "I feel so much better than I did a while back. I feel like I've come a long way."

**O:**   Pt. seen for discharge planning from Medicare A → Medicare B. Pt. seen 15/20 tx sessions from SOC. Pt. illness prevented attending 5 sessions. Pt. seen for ADL retraining, toileting, functional transfer training, ↑ AROM and strength.
Pt. level of function at D/C as follows:

| Goals: | Initial: | D/C: |
|---|---|---|
| Dressing UE ⓘ | Min Ⓐ for balance | Set-up |
| LE ⓘ | Mod Ⓐ for balance | Set-up c̄ CGA for standing to don pants and panties |
| Bathing UE ⓘ | Min Ⓐ | ⓘ UE |
| LE ⓘ | Min Ⓐ | ⓘ using long handled sponge |

*Transfers*
| | | |
|---|---|---|
| *Sit ⇆ supine* ① | *SBA* Ⓐ | *SBA* |
| *Sit ⇆ stand* ① | *Min* Ⓐ | *SBA* |
| *Stand ⇆ w/c or toilet* | *CGA c̄ mod verbal cues* | *SBA* |

| | | |
|---|---|---|
| | *Shoulder abd-65° (strength 2)* | *Shoulder abd 90° (strength 3)* |
| *AROM-WFL* | *Shoulder flex-55° (strength 2)* | *Shoulder flex-60° (strength 3)* |
| | *Elbow-0-125 (strength 3-)* | *Elbow-WFL (strength 4)* |

**A:**    *Pt. exhibited an increase in AROM and strength. Pt. has met bathing and hygiene goals. Dressing and transfer goals partially met. Resident is continuing to make progress and would benefit from further OT intervention to increase UE strength and activity tolerance to perform ADLs ① and meet all goals.*

**P:**    *Discharged from skilled OT 2° change of status from Medicare A → Medicare B. Request physician's orders to reevaluate under Medicare B. Upon physician's orders, recommend skilled OT intervention 3 x week to increase activity tolerance and strength to perform ADLs ①.*

Carrie Student, OTR/L

# WORKSHEET 10-5

## *Discharge Summary #1 (SOAP Format)*

Use this worksheet to determine whether the summary on pages 121 and 122 meet the AOTA criteria.

| Criteria | Compliance |
|---|---|
| What interventions were used? | |
| How many treatment sessions were there? | |
| How did the consumer respond? | |
| To what degree were the short- and long-term functional goals achieved? | |
| How does functional status prior to therapy compare to status at discharge? | |
| Is there evidence that a home program was or was not given? Is it attached? | |
| What is schedule and specific plan for follow-up? | |
| What are the recommendations pertaining to the consumer's future needs? | |

Adapted from *Elements of Clinical Documentation* (Revision) (AOTA, 1998a)

# Rehabilitation Center Occupational Therapy
# Discharge Summary

**Date:** 2/19/99          **Time:** 3:00 PM

### Course of Rehabilitation:

*Pt. seen 20/20 sessions from SOC on 1/25/99. Skilled instruction in adaptive techniques for ADLs provided. Pt. progress was good and she met all tx. goals. Pt. now requires SBA in all transfers, lower body ADLs, upper body ADLs, grooming/hygiene. She is Ⓘ in toileting. Pt. also requires SBA in feeding after setup. Dressing from armchair with wheeled walker, set-up only but SBA for standing and to pull pants up over hips. Bathing is SBA with min Ⓐ w/c ⇆ shower using tub bench.*

### Patient Education:

*Recommendations for additional adaptive equipment and modifications to home discussed with pt. and caregiver. Pt. and caregiver were instructed in home exercise program of Thera-Band, free weights, wands, and other activities to choose from for Ⓑ UE strengthening. HEP discussed with pt. and pt. demonstrated ability to perform exercises correctly.*

### Discharge Recommendations/Referrals:

*Discharge with home caregiver. Continue home exercise program. Assistive equipment recommended—walker basket and reacher holder for walker. Pt. already has wheeled walker, reacher, dressing stick, sock aid, long shoehorn, and functional bathroom equipment, and has demonstrated ability to use these correctly and safely. Pt. will be seen in outpatient PT. No direct OT services are recommended at this time.*

Paul Howard, OTR/L

# WORKSHEET 10-6

## *Discharge Summary #2 (Facility Form)*

**Use this worksheet to determine whether the summary on page 125 meets the AOTA criteria.**

| Criteria | Compliance |
|---|---|
| What interventions were used? | |
| How many treatment sessions were there? | |
| How did the consumer respond? | |
| To what degree were the short- and long-term functional goals achieved? | |
| How does functional status prior to therapy compare to status at discharge? | |
| Is there evidence that a home program was or was not given? Is it attached? | |
| What is schedule and specific plan for follow-up? | |
| What are the recommendations pertaining to the consumer's future needs? | |

Adapted from *Elements of Clinical Documentation* (Revision) (AOTA, 1998a)

# CHAPTER 11
## Documentation in Different Practice Settings

In this chapter we will examine documentation practices in three different practice settings: mental health, the public schools, and long-term care facilities. Each of these has some requirements that are specific to the setting or the primary payment source. Documentation for these settings is different in some ways from the examples you have learned so far.

## Documentation in Mental Health

If your first job is in a mental health setting, you might think that nothing you have been taught about documentation applies. Problems, goals, and interventions are often multidisciplinary and may be written in a different format from what you have learned. The language used in the documentation will seem less specific. Also, intervention is provided in a milieu environment involving a multitude of mental health professionals all working toward the same goals with the patient. Occupational therapy services are often included in a treatment service designated as adjunctive therapy, activity therapy, or expressive therapy that may include therapeutic recreation specialists, music therapists, art therapists, and dance therapists. The roles often overlap and there is a blurring of professional identities. The reimbursement is usually not discipline specific in these types of settings, and therapy services are usually inclusive in a room rate for the facility.

One of the exceptions is geriatric psychiatric mental health units or partial hospitals where the patients are usually insured through Medicare. The documentation is similar to inpatient Medicare requirements but the types of intervention covered include psychiatric occupational therapy services as well as self-care interventions (Lopes, 1998). As occupational therapy services become more community-based, the reimbursement patterns change and the funding may not be client specific but service specific. The documentation may be based more on program outcomes and population-based services (Ramsey & Auerbach, 1997). Even so, the documentation of services provided in community based programs should reflect the principles and concepts used for OT assessments, plans of intervention, and records of progress of recipients of services. This means that your documentation should be objective and measurable and focused on occupational performance.

**Initial evaluation reports** often reflect the disciplines included in activity therapy rather than each discipline, thus losing the some of the professional identity of occupational therapy. From the initial evaluation, the occupational therapist contributes to the treatment team's efforts to compile a list of problem statements.

### Multidisciplinary Treatment Plans in Mental Health Care

Treatment plans in mental health are usually multidisciplinary. The therapeutic milieu is considered to be critical in caring for patients who have mental illnesses, and the individualized treatment plan (ITP) in a mental health setting is a contract for change between the patient and all members of the treatment team. After each individual discipline assesses the patient's needs and strengths, the team meets to formulate a list of the problems to be addressed. From this problem list, each individual discipline suggests goals, objectives and interventions for treatment within that discipline. All goals, objectives, and interventions for each discipline involved in the patient or client's care are written into one comprehensive plan.

If major problems or concerns have been identified in the evaluation, they must be documented somewhere on the ITP. It is critical that the plan is formulated by all who will be participating in it including the client and all staff who will be providing any part of the treatment. Multidisciplinary plans can often be quite long, since they are compilations of several different disciplines. These plans are similar to those developed by teams in a rehabilitation setting or school setting, but differ in that all staff are working toward the same goals but through different interventions.

The plan must be easily understood by the patient or client and there must be some indication that the patient is in agreement with the plan, as required by most accrediting agencies. This is usually accomplished by the patient's signature on the bottom of the plan.

A multidisciplinary plan may contain fewer objectives per goal than a discipline specific plan. Success in writing a multidisciplinary treatment plan depends on:

1.     The involvement of the client (and family, if they are a part of the client's present life).
2.     The willingness of each member of the treatment team to cooperate in a coordinated effort to carry out specific interventions.
3.     Regular evaluation of the effectiveness of the plan and changes in direction in interventions that have not been effective.

Functional problem statements in a mental health practice setting are traditionally divided into two parts, as noted in *Chapter 2: Documenting the Treatment Process in Occupational Therapy*. The problem itself is stated in one or two words, such as "depressed mood", "noncompliant behavior", "suicidal ideation," or "alcohol withdrawal." The behavioral manifestations that follow give the performance areas and performance components. For example:

> **Problem:** *Chemical dependence*
> **Behavioral manifestations:** *Mark has been using alcohol since age 12 with increasing frequency over the last year, and also admits to using cocaine, "crystal," opium, and marijuana; resulting in a failed marriage, loss of two jobs, and involvement with the criminal justice system.*

> **Problem:** *Drug use*
> **Behavioral manifestations:** *Kathy uses marijuana on a daily basis until she becomes high, thus depression and verbal altercations ensue at home and in school.*

> **Problem:** *Noncompliant behavior*
> **Behavioral manifestations:** *Patient disobeys foster parents by running away, refusal to follow rules or requests, and engaging in sexual activity, resulting in six foster home placements in the past 4 years.*

> **Problem:** *Suicide risk*
> **Behavioral manifestations:** *During the week prior to admission, the patient verbalized suicidal ideation, stating that life was no longer worth living. On the day of admission he purchased a handgun.*

**Goals and objectives** are often interdisciplinary, contributing to the role defusion and lack of professional identity. Each discipline works on the same goals, using its individual treatment strategies. Occupational therapists in an inpatient mental health practice setting must decide what constitutes an instrumental ADL. Answering this question is one of the challenges of working in a setting that requires the team to document its ability to work together to provide a therapeutic milieu. Is remaining sober, decreasing family conflict, or keeping a marriage together an IADL? In addition, goals and objectives are often selected from computer programs or provided on preprinted sheets for each problem, as illustrated later in this chapter. In community settings, occupational therapy goals can be related more easily and clearly to ADL functioning.

**Interventions** are usually focused on the goals of the milieu setting, and those specific to activity therapy may be addressed by activity therapy in general and not specific to the disciplines represented by the activity therapy staff. The choice of interventions may depend largely upon what treatment groups are being provided by the facility, with the ability to individualize intervention strategies within the groups themselves. Selecting meaningful treatment interventions can be an interesting challenge. For example, most patients may attend communication groups, but within those groups, you as an occupational therapist are able to customize the way you choose to increase communication skills for each individual patient. A good therapist learns to individualize goals for each patient in the group while still providing for the needs of the group as a whole.

When planning treatment, the client's assets (good verbal skills, intelligence, etc.) will be the tools that the client has to use in overcoming her problems. A "strength" in this context is an ability, a skill, or an interest that the client has used in the past or has the potential for doing. Assets can include such things as the client's interests (enjoys playing music), abilities (writes well), relationship skills (has a good relationship with her father), and social support systems (minister keeps in contact). Assets may also be past abilities that the treatment team wants to encourage as treatment progresses (Jane was physically active before she became ill). Some interests (enjoys going to bars on weekends) may not be assets.

## Treatment Notes

Formal treatment notes are rarely written in an inpatient mental health setting, although incidents are documented. One of the exceptions is geriatric psychiatric inpatient and partial hospitalization units where the patients are usually Medicare insured. In these settings, the documentation follows Medicare requirements.

Progress notes are usually written weekly, and the occupational therapist makes treatment notes for his own use in compiling the progress notes. However, if a patient with a mental health diagnosis is seen in home health, the Medicare standards for home health that require treatment notes for each visit apply.

When you begin thinking in the language of mental health, like "brightened affect" or "less delusional," or "improved mood," it is easy to begin letting go of your ability to think in more objective and measurable terms. If you think about it, though, there are always clues that you are using to decide just exactly why you think the patient's affect is brighter or his mood is improved. Perhaps you are seeing him smile more frequently, or initiate conversation more often, or respond to your "hello" by making eye contact. Perhaps she takes less time to get up and dressed in the morning, or is more easily persuaded to attend OT. These indicators are all measurable, and it is very helpful to the treatment team if you are able to report your observations in measurable and behavioral terms.

The trend toward role diffusion is making it more difficult for occupational therapists to document OT as a service that offers good value for the dollars spent in mental health care. As resources shrink and costs expand, we need to focus on documenting functional changes that are cost-effective and meaningful to both the payer and to the consumer. As noted in Chapter 1, we are in the business of solving problems in occupational performance, and there are a myriad of occupational performance deficits present in the lives of people who have mental illness and chemical dependency. If we want to remain a viable force in inpatient mental health settings and if we want to continue to address the psychosocial issues related to physical dysfunction, we need to be able to document what we do that is unique. We need to be clear about the way our services change functional outcomes (Kannenberg, 1998).

The use of a multidisciplinary plan allows for effective utilization and coordination of all available services in order to maximize the client's potential for meaningful change. The plan provided on the following pages is an example of a multidisciplinary treatment plan from an inpatient adolescent mental health setting. It is common for the client to have several problems that are being addressed, with each problem listed on a separate page. In this kind of plan, OT is integrated into the multidisciplinary plan in several different places, depending on the problem being discussed.

# Behavioral Health Center Master Treatment Plan

Name: Tina W.
Problem #: 1

Page: 1
Date: 12/27/98

Problem: Tina states that she does not have any good feelings about herself and that she has considered suicide, resulting in safety concerns.

Goal: Tina will verbalize both positive feelings about herself and the absence of suicidal ideation by D/C on 1/31/99.

| Start Date | Measurable Objectives | Exp. Date Achieved | Method of Treatment | Freq. | Responsible Person |
|---|---|---|---|---|---|
| 12/27/98 | 1. Tina will identify areas of her life that she feels are inadequate and discuss with primary therapist. | 12/30/98 | Individual Therapy | 2x wk. | S. Young, M.Ed. |
| 12/27/98 | 2. Tina will identify five areas about herself that are positive and discuss in groups and in individual therapy. | 1/7/99 | Individual Therapy | 2x wk. | S. Young, M.Ed. |
| | | | Discussion with nursing staff | Daily | A. Smith, R.N. |
| | | | Occupational Therapy | 3x wk. | S.Borcherding, OTR |
| | | | Emotions Anonymous | 3x wk. | A. Smith, R.N. |
| 12/27/98 | 3. Tina will discuss areas of her life that are positive and negative with peers and receive feedback in group therapy, E.A., and OT. | 1/14/99 | Group Therapy | 5x wk. | P. Alton, M.Ed. |
| | | | Emotions Anonymous | 3x wk. | A. Smith, R.N. |
| | | | Communication Skills Group | 1x wk. | S.Borcherding, OTR |
| | | | Step Study | 3x wk. | S. Williams, BSW |
| 12/27/98 | 4. Tina will select three new activities that she feels would be beneficial to her life and compose a plan for continuing these after discharge. | 1/20/99 | Occupational Therapy will introduce Tina to new leisure skill | 3x wk. | S. Matsuda, COTA |
| 12/27/98 | 5. Tina will discuss her needs, assets, and plans with her mother. | 1/20/99 | Individual therapy to formulate list of needs and a plan | 2x wk. | S. Young, M.Ed. |
| | | | Family therapy to discuss plans and needs with mother | 1x wk. | S. Young, M.Ed. |
| 12/27/98 | 6. Tina will complete all school assignments and earn passing grades in all subjects. | 1/30/99 | Education staff will provide positive feedback for good schoolwork | 5x wk. | M. Green |

# Behavioral Health Center Master Treatment Plan

Page: 2

**Name:** Tina W.                                                        **Date:** 12/27/98
**Problem #:** 2
**Problem:** Tina expresses her anger at her mother by choosing the "wrong" boyfriend, lying, and running away, resulting in her removal from the home.
**Goal:** Tina will verbally express anger to her mother by D/C on 1/31/99.

| Start Date | Measurable Objectives | Exp. Date Achieved | Method of Treatment | Freq. | Responsible Person |
|---|---|---|---|---|---|
| 12/27/98 | 1. Tina will attend health center groups that provide educational material on dealing with feelings. | 12/30/98 | Psycho. Ed. Emotions Anonymous | 3x wk. 3x wk. | M. Eveker, RN A. Smith, RN |
| | | | Occupational Therapy | 1x wk. | S. Borcherding, OTR |
| | | | Group Therapy | 5x wk. | P. Alton, M.Ed. |
| 12/27/98 | 2. Tina will discuss past ways of dealing with anger with primary therapist. | 1/7/99 | Individual Therapy | 2x wk. | S. Young, M.Ed. |
| 12/27/98 | 3. Tina will list three alternate ways of dealing with her anger toward her mother. | 1/14/99 | Appropriate way of dealing with anger will be discussed in individual therapy and Occupational Therapy | 3x wk. | S. Young, M.Ed. S. Borcherding, OTR |
| 12/27/98 | 4. Tina will practice alternative ways of dealing with her anger. | 1/20/99 | All staff will remind Tina to practice her alternative methods when she becomes angry | Daily | S. Borcherding, OTR A. Smith, R.N. |
| 12/27/98 | 5. Tina will enter into a behavior contract with her mother regarding how anger is to be expressed and received in their household. | 1/20/99 | Individual therapist will assist family in writing the contract | 2x wk. | S. Young, M.Ed. |

Some mental health centers use prepackaged treatment planning sheets or mix-and-match computerized programs from which problem, goal, and intervention statements can be selected. In a mix-and-match program, the computer provides prompts from which the therapist selects the problem statements, goals, objectives, and treatment interventions that will be used for the individual patient.

When using prepackaged treatment planning sheets, the problems are expressed briefly, e.g., *depressed mood, drug abuse, suicide risk,* and the behavioral manifestations that apply to the individual patient are written in.

There is a list of long-term goals, or **outcomes**, such as these:

*Patient will report the absence of suicidal ideation.*

*Patient will identify three new coping strategies to use when he feels the urge to use drugs.*

All members of the interdisciplinary treatment team work on these goals while the patient is in the therapeutic milieu. The wisdom of using multidisciplinary goals without a strong functional component for occupational therapy practice has been seriously questioned by therapists who practice in mental health settings (Kannenberg, 1998). The question of exactly what constitutes an IADL in mental health care has not been definitively answered at this time.

On a prepackaged form there is a list of potential interventions that would also be addressed by the treatment team. Interventions might include such strategies as the following:
- Evaluate the patient
- Encourage patient to express emotions
- Teach new coping skills
- Encourage the patient to verbalize alternatives to previous coping strategies
- Assist the patient to develop a discharge plan that will prevent recurrence

Each discipline implements the interventions in its own way. In relation to the five intervention strategies listed above, the occupational therapist does an OT evaluation to determine problems in occupational performance areas. He uses OT media and OT groups to encourage the patient to express emotions. He uses OT media and OT groups to teach new coping skills and to encourage the patient to verbalize alternatives. He helps the patient make a plan for any of the occupational performance areas that had been a part of the previous problem. Social work adapts the same treatment interventions to individual and group therapy, and nursing implements the interventions on the unit. In this situation, there are sheets provided for each goal that are commonly used. It is individualized to the patient by stating behavioral manifestations of the problem, and by adding and deleting outcomes and/or interventions.

An example of such a prepackaged treatment planning sheet for alcohol dependence follows. It is provided only as an example of what might be seen in practice. **This does not represent a suggestion for best practice in preparing treatment plans.**

# Behavioral Health Center Multidisciplinary Treatment Plan

**Problem #:**              **Problem name:** Alcohol Dependence    **Date Identified:**
**Behavioral Manifestations:**

| Desired Outcomes | Target Date | Date Achieved |
|---|---|---|
| 1. Pt. will verbally acknowledge that alcohol use has been a problem and will state an intent to abstain from alcohol use. | | |
| 2. Pt. will have developed at least three new ways to deal with stress and will have demonstrated use of these. | | |
| 3. Pt. will have an aftercare plan in place. | | |
| 4. Pt. will have established a 5 day period of sobriety and of attending AA meetings daily. | | |
| 5. | | |

| Treatment Interventions | Staff Responsible |
|---|---|
| 1. Evaluation of the patient's alcohol intake and use patterns.<br>2. Provide individual, group, and family therapy.<br>3. Education, re: the disease model of chemical dependency.<br>4. Provide opportunities to express feelings.<br>5. Teach coping skills.<br>6. Assist patient to restructure environmental situations.<br>7. Evaluate and teach relationship skills.<br>8. Facilitate peer confrontation and feedback.<br>9. Introduce social/leisure activities that do not include alcohol.<br>10. | |

I agree with this plan.

_____     _____

*Patient's Signature*                                      *Date*

## Critical Care Pathways in Mental Health

As length of stay has shortened for psychiatric diagnoses, some mental health settings have begun using critical care pathways as well as the standardized treatment planning programs discussed earlier. Critical care pathways in mental health are multidisciplinary and are conceptually the same as those in rehabilitation. The plan for the consumer's care for each day for each discipline is preplanned in order to make the most efficient use of staff time during the short length of stay, while still making sure the consumer's needs are met.

# Documentation in School-Based Practice

When your caseload consists of children in the public schools, you learn a slightly different language for the same concepts. You now work under a treatment plan called an Individualized Education Plan (IEP), and you write problems, goals, and interventions focused on behaviors and skills the child needs to be successful in school. The IEP is a multidisciplinary plan compiled by therapists, teachers, and parents. Based on an assessment from each discipline, it details the current problems, goals, and interventions for the child in all areas including OT for the current school year. The treatment principles and concepts are basically the same—only the language is different. That language difference, however, is very important.

The **treatment plan** is multidisciplinary, and is called an Individual Education Plan. The IEP is also specific to treatment of the child's educational and classroom problems and needs.

**Functional problem statements** are exclusively problems of occupational performance in the educational setting, even though the child may have many deficits in other areas of life.

**Goal statements** are written for the duration of the school year, rather than using a timeline for each goal. In this setting, goals for the school year are called "objectives." Sometimes the format is slightly different, with a "criteria" added to make the goal specific. It is very important not to set goals for performance components in this setting.

**Interventions** are specific to the educational setting as well, even though the child may also need treatment for problems in other areas of occupational performance.

Since an IEP can be quite long, the one provided here has been condensed from its original 26 pages to show only those aspects that are representative or most pertinent to OT.

# Schools—Special Services Department
# Individualized Education Plan

**Student:** Truman T.  **Date of Birth:** 9/17/83  **Parents:** Linda and Ellis T.
**Teacher:** Mary Ellen W.  **Case Manager:** Sharon Y.  **IEP Conference Date:** 5/23/99
**Annual Review Date:** 5/23/00  **Duration of Services:** 1 year  **Initial Placement Date:** 9/27/98
**Service Model:** Regular education: 100 minutes    initiated 5/24/99    ending 5/24/00
                        Special education: 1550 minutes    initiated 5/24/99    ending 5/24/00
**Related Services:** Occupational therapy, physical therapy, adaptive PE, special transportation
**Placement:** Self-contained classroom
**Assistive Devices:** Glasses    **Physical Education:** Adaptive PE
**Special Transition Services Needed:** Instruction, related services, daily living skills
**Specialized Materials:** Easel, bookstand for academic and fine motor activities, enlarged monitor
                        for computer, pencil grip
**Notification of Progress:** Parents will be given a copy of the goals and progress four times per
                        year with the report card.
**Present Level of Performance:** Truman has been diagnosed with cerebral palsy (quadriplegic), developmental delays, and visual difficulties. He wears glasses and needs written work enlarged. He has a history of ear infections and has bilateral PE tubes in place. Truman displays low muscle tone, with compensatory fluctuating increased tone upon movement. Fine motor skills include spasticity noted in both arms on passive range of motion. Grip strength has improved, but bilateral tasks remain difficult due to poor lateral trunk control. He requires minimal to moderate assistance to hold his arms in different positions simultaneously. He requires moderate assistance to use scissors. His speech and language skills are commensurate with his intellectual functioning, in the mentally handicapped range of abilities. The WISC II suggests that his general information and verbal reasoning skills are at a 6 year age level. Non-verbal abilities are at about the same level. Truman shows difficulty with visual-spatial abilities, visual-motor integration, gross-motor production, and visual-perceptual processing. Vocabulary is low. He has a relative strength in short-term auditory memory and ability to sequence small bits of information. His ability to perceive patterns and relations is impaired, as is his neuropsychological processing of tactile stimuli. His adaptive behavior is below average. Current level of functioning is the 1.0-1.5 grade level. Reading comprehension and spelling ability are age equivalent 6-0, with math computation at an age level of 7-0. Adaptive functioning suggests an age equivalent of approximately 5-0 years. He is able to use a telephone in an emergency, look both ways before crossing the street, and get a drink of water from a tap unassisted. Progress has been made in adaptive functioning, but significant deficits remain in regard to toileting, dressing, functional mobility, and food preparation skills. No significant behavioral difficulties exist either at school or at home. Truman has limited interactions with peers, and limited participation in the regular classroom. He attends technology lab twice a week with a student aide. He works best on a 1-1 basis for 15 to 20 minute intervals in a situation where auditory distractions are limited.

**Annual Goal #1:** Truman will show school/homework responsibilities
**Implementer:** Special Education Teacher

> *Short-term Objective #1: Truman will be responsible for homework in different areas of study at least 2 times weekly.*
> *Evaluation Procedure: Observation*

> *Short-term Objective #2: Truman will be responsible for taking notebook home and returning it the following day. Homework assignments consisting of spelling words, reading and math sheets, counting change, and time worksheets will be listed in this book.*

**Annual Goal #2:** Truman will improve skills in adaptive physical education
**Implementer:** Adaptive PE teacher/paraprofessional

*Short-term Objective:* Truman will sit up.
*Evaluation Procedure:* Observation          *Criteria:* Without being reminded for ½ hour

**Annual Goal #3:** Truman will use computers in the classroom and computer lab
**Implementer:** Special Education Teacher/Paraprofessionals

*Short-term Objective:* Truman will use computers with assistance.
*Evaluation Procedure:* Observation          *Criteria:* 80% accuracy

**Annual Goal #4:** Truman will improve math skills.
**Implementer:** Special Education Teacher

*Short-term Objective:* Given a clock dial, Truman will say the time to the 5-minute interval.
*Evaluation Procedure:* Daily work          *Criteria:* 80% accuracy 3 of 4 tracking days

**Annual Goal # 5:** Improve fine motor for greater success with classroom related activities
**Implementer:** Occupational Therapist

*Short-term Objective #1:* Truman will cut 8" using adaptive scissors with minimal assistance to adjust grasp and paper position.
*Evaluation Procedure:* Daily work          *Criteria:* 75% accuracy

*Short-term Objective #2:* Truman will type 10 spelling words on an adaptive computer keyboard using isolated index finger movements.
*Evaluation Procedure:* Daily work          *Criteria:* No more than two errors

**Annual Goal #6:** Increase visual motor skills for greater success in academic work
**Implementer:** Occupational Therapist

*Short-term Objective:* Truman will demonstrate good attention to task and visual motor skills in order to sort 15 small items.
*Evaluation procedure:* Observation          *Criteria:* Within 90 seconds with minimal verbal cues and 75% accuracy

**Annual Goal #7:** Truman will exhibit increased functional motor skills in the school environment
**Implementer:** Physical Therapist

*Short-term Objective:* Sitting on a box, Truman will lean forward and sit upright picking up objects from the floor.
*Evaluation Procedure:* Observation          *Criteria:* Eight times with 50% assistance from therapist after 10 consecutive sessions

**Least Restrictive Environment:** Self-contained special education classroom
**Related Services:** Occupational therapy, Transportation, Assistive technology, Language therapy
**Will student be receiving services in school closest to home?** __X__ yes          ____ no
**IEP services that cannot be provided in the regular classroom:** Math, reading, written expression, listening comprehension, language, physical therapy, occupational therapy, transition

Factors for consideration of removal:
>  **Nature and severity of the disability**
>> Difficulty performing activity of daily living at an age-appropriate level
>> Receptive/expressive language skills interfere with communication
>> Easily distracted/frequently off task
>
>  **Diverse learning style of the student**
>> Requires highly structured small-group setting
>> Lacks social/behavioral skills for participation in regular classroom
>> Requires exposure to experiences not available in regular classroom
>> Individualized instruction
>> Increased drill/practice to master skills
>> Immediate corrective feedback
>> Additional time to complete task
>> Positive rewards
>
>  **Inability to engage appropriately with other students**
>> Requires inordinate amount of teacher time
>> Learning styles cannot be addressed in regular classroom
>> Expressive language skills inadequate for classroom participation
>> Receptive language skills interfere with academic progress

## Occupational Therapy Evaluation/Progress Report

This 13-year-old male has received occupational therapy services throughout his school years with treatment most recently three times weekly for 45-minute sessions to work on improving fine motor and visual motor skills. Truman lives with his parents who are very supportive, active in his care, and motivated to see him succeed to his highest potential. He has many adaptations in his home to promote independence and assist caregivers.

Truman presents as friendly and kind, and wanting to please. He apologizes when he is unable to complete what is asked of him, although at times he will complain of being too tired to complete a task. He is very social and gets along with both peers and adults. Due to his cognitive limitations, standard testing would not give valid results. For this reason, observation of functioning has been used.

## Fine Motor

Low muscle tone with moderate spasticity noted Ⓑ upon PROM. Elbows are contracted by calcium deposits to -30° Ⓡ and -40° Ⓛ. Truman is Ⓡ hand dominant. Grip strength Ⓡ is from 15-20# and Ⓛ from 8-16# in the past year. Truman has difficulty with Ⓑ tasks due to lateral trunk instability that requires use of one hand to stabilize himself. He has a hypersensitive startle reflex that kicks in when he feels like he is losing his balance. He has been working on disassociating arms so that he can use one for movement while the other is doing a different movement, and requires moderate assistance to do this. He is able to open a soda can after the seal has been broken with extra time given. He requires verbal reminders 75% of the time to use his Ⓛ arm to stabilize an object with one hand while manipulating it with the other. He requires moderate assist for scissor use and requires assistance to stabilize the paper. His arms become stiffened as he recruits all his muscle fibers to hold on to scissors and paper. Despite this, he has made great gains in scissor use over the past year.

## Visual Motor/Visual Perception

Truman has severe visual problems and needs adaptive equipment to compensate for his visual deficits, including a large screen monitor and adaptive keyboard with the letters in alphabetical order. For future use, an adapted keyboard with enlarged letters in the regular order is recommended. He is able to use the mouse to move coins on the screen into a narrow slot with 75% accuracy.

Truman has a poor ability to track objects and poor ocular motor control. It is hard to tell what he can see, because he often guesses at responses. He is able to find objects in the classroom and to maneuver his wheelchair around obstacles. He has demonstrated great gains in visual motor paper and pencil skills, progressing from the inability to draw vertical and horizontal lines to the ability to copy circles, squares, and triangles with moderate assistance and dot-to-dot guides. Adapted equipment (vertical slant board and enlarged writing utensils) are needed for writing.

## Gross Motor

Overall low tone with compensatory fluctuating increased tone upon movement. Specific exercises are performed daily as a part of adaptive PE.

## Sensory Integration

No sensory defensiveness or unusual sensory behaviors.

## Self-Help

**Functional Mobility:** Able to wheel his chair within school environment with extra time.
**Feeding:** He generally chooses finger foods but has demonstrated ability to use utensils with built up handles.
**Toileting, Dressing (coat), Wheelchair Positioning:** Requires moderate assistance for these tasks. He is very private with his toileting and prefers males to assist him. He often slides forward in his wheelchair and has difficulty sitting upright and righting himself once he has leaned to the side. He would benefit from a wheelchair back that provides some lateral support and a cushion that will decrease the slide forward.

## Summary

Truman has made great gains in fine motor strength and visual motor skills over the past year. Harrington rod placement greatly increased his ability to interact within the school environment. He seems motivated to succeed. Strengths include his supportive family, his motivation, his general good health, and emotional stability. Areas of concern continue to be his muscle weakness with compensatory abnormal movement patterns and visual motor/visual perceptual difficulties. If daily strengthening continues to be provided by school staff, Truman would benefit from OT at a decreased rate to focus on monitoring and training staff to assist him with exercise, visual motor, and bilateral coordination tasks.

## Recommendations

Continue OT services twice weekly for 45-minute sessions to work on areas of concern listed above. Continue use of adaptive equipment listed above. Begin transitional planning for skills necessary after high school.

Linda P. Eagle, OTR/L

## Documentation in Skilled Nursing Facilities in Long-Term Care

Most patients who receive therapy services in long-term care settings at skilled nursing facilities are covered by Medicare, and documentation is usually done using specialized Medicare forms.

When a patient is first admitted, a multidisciplinary evaluation called the Minimum Data Set (MDS) is used to determine the level of care needed. For ease and efficiency, each discipline may be assigned a specific part of the MDS to complete. Facilities may vary in how ADL sections are divided between occupational therapy and nursing. Patients are then divided into Resource Utilization Groupings (RUGs) according to how much care they need. If this process is done improperly, the patient will not be able to get the level of care needed. Also, inaccurate assessments and predictions about rehabilitation potential may result in the facility not being able to be reimbursed for care that is provided beyond what was indicated on the MDS.

The initial assessment for a Medicare patient is recorded on a Medicare 700 form (Figure 11-1), and contains a history, any medical complications that will impact treatment, the reason for referral, and the level of function at the start of care. As you can see in the example that follows, there is very limited space available for recording the initial evaluation report. The treatment plan is divided into two sections. There is a small space to record "Plan of Treatment Functional Goals" (short-term goals) and the "Outcome" or long-term goals. There is a separate small space for interventions. The example that follows shows the information recorded in the amount of space that is available.

Progress notes are done monthly on a Medicare 701 form (Figure 11-2), which provides equally small spaces for the reason(s) for continuing treatment for an additional billing period. In this section you must clarify your goals and document the reason for continuing skilled occupational therapy.

Occupational therapists working in skilled nursing facilities in long-term care settings must learn to be very concise, providing all the necessary information in the fewest words possible. Some therapists have learned to manage the space constraints by using a specialized computer program that contains the form and reduces the font to the smallest size that is readable. However, some therapists are in situations in which they need to hand write the information into the space provided while still recording everything that is required.

| DEPARTMENT OF HEALTH AND HUMAN SERVICES<br>HEALTH CARE FINANCING ADMINISTRATION | Part A    Part B    Other<br>Specify | FORM APPROVED<br>OMB NO. 0938-0227 |
|---|---|---|

## PLAN OF TREATMENT FOR OUTPATIENT REHABILITATION (COMPLETE FOR INITIAL CLAIMS ONLY)

| 1. PATIENT'S LAST NAME<br>XXXXXXXXXX | FIRST NAME    M.I<br>XXXXXX     X. | 2. PROVIDER NO.<br>XXXXX | 3. HICN<br>XXXXX |
|---|---|---|---|
| 4. PROVIDER NAME<br>Provident Rehabilitation | 5. MEDICAL RECORD NO.<br>(Optional) | 6. ONSET DATE<br>3/23/99 | 7. SOC. DATE<br>5/5/99 |
| 8. TYPE:<br>☐ PT ☐ OT ☐ SLP ☐ CR<br>☐ RT ☐ PS ☐ SN ☐ SW | 9. PRIMARY DIAGNOSIS<br>(Pertinent medical DX)<br>pneumonia, Parkinson's Disease | 10. TREATMENT DIAGNOSIS<br>Decrease in function 780.9 | 11. VISITS FROM SOC. |

| 12. PLAN OF TREATMENT FUNCTIONAL GOALS | PLAN |
|---|---|
| GOALS (Short-Term)<br>2 wks: Pt. will be: 1. SBA in bed mobility with adaptations to use bedside commode. 2. Ⓘ c̄ sit↔stand transfers to bed and toilet. 3. Able to ambulate using walker with SBA for safety↔bathroom. 4. Propel self in w/c Ⓘ ½ way to dining room. 5. Min Ⓐ dressing.<br><br>OUTCOME (Long-Term)<br>6 wks: In order to perform ADLs at home, pt. will be: 1. Ⓘ in mobility & transfers. 2. Ⓘ in toileting using bedside commode or bathroom. 3. Ⓘ in w/c mobility. 4. Ⓘ in dressing and bathing c̄ set-up. | ADL retraining<br><br>Transfer training<br><br>Functional Mobility training<br><br>Safety education |

| 13. SIGNATURE (professional establishing POC including prof. designation)<br><br>**I CERTIFY THE NEED FOR THESE SERVICES FURNISHED UNDER THIS PLAN OF TREATMENT AND WHILE UNDER MY CARE**   N/A | 14. FREQ/DURATION (e.g. 3/Wk x 4 Wk.)<br>5/Wk x 2 Wk   then 3/Wk x 4 Wk |
|---|---|
|  | 17. CERTIFICATION<br>FROM   5/5/99     THROUGH 5/30/99   ☐ N/A |
| 15. PHYSICIAN'S SIGNATURE     16. DATE | 18. ON FILE (Print/type physician's name) |

| 20. INITIAL ASSESSMENT (History, medical complications, level of function at start of care. Reason for referral) | 19. PRIOR HOSPITALIZATION<br>FROM     TO     ☐ N/A |
|---|---|

Pt. is 73 y/o/f who lived alone and did accounting work until hospitalized for pneumonia 3/23/99 and transferred to this facility 5/1/99. Pt. states she wants to move to her daughter's home and be Ⓘ in transfers and mobility as in the past. Medical Hx. and complications include Parkinson's disease and frequent falls. Prior to her illness, pt. was Ⓘ in bed mobility, ADLs, meal & tax preparations. Pt. was referred by nursing on 5/5/99 2° to pt. feeling better and being able to benefit from therapy. Cognition: alert and oriented x3; uses phone to direct family and clients from bed. ADL tasks: Pt. mod Ⓐ in bathing and dressing due to fatigue from illness and complications of inactivity and Parkinson's disease. Pt. feeds self after set up. Mobility: Pt. max Ⓐ in bed mobility supine to sit; mod Ⓐ in transfers and requires SBA assistance to ambulate in room using wheeled walker for safety and is propelled in w/c outside her room by staff due to fatigue, balance and ambulation difficulties. AROM is WFL but pt. is slow to initiate movements. Strength is 4/5 in Ⓑ UEs. Grip strength is 10# on Ⓡ, 8# on Ⓛ. Pt. is motivated and rehab potential is excellent for discharge to daughter's home with caregiver and possible home health or meals-on-wheels assistance. Pt. would benefit from skilled OT instruction in safe use of assistive devices, transfer techniques, and home evaluation before discharge.

| 21. FUNCTIONAL LEVEL (End of billing period)    PROGRESS REPORT    ☐ CONTINUE SERVICES    OR    ☐ DC SERVICES |
|---|

| 22. SERVICE DATES |
|---|
| FROM             THROUGH |

Figure 11-1. Department of Health and Human Services Health Care Financing Administration Form HCFA-700.

| DEPARTMENT OF HEALTH AND HUMAN SERVICES<br>HEALTH CARE FINANCING ADMINISTRATION | Part A    Part B    Other<br>Specify | FORM APPROVED<br>OMB NO. 0938-0227 | |
|---|---|---|---|

**UPDATED PLAN OF TREATMENT FOR OUTPATIENT REHABILITATION** *(COMPLETE FOR INTERIM TO DISCHARGE CLAIMS. PHOTOCOPY OF HCFA-700 OR 701 IS REQUIRED)*

| 1. PATIENT'S LAST NAME<br>XXXXXXXXXX | FIRST NAME          M.I<br>XXXXXX               X. | 2. PROVIDER NO.<br>XXXXX | 3. HICN<br>XXXXX |
|---|---|---|---|
| 4. PROVIDER NAME<br>Provident Rehabilitation | 5. MEDICAL RECORD NO.<br>*(Optional)* | 6. ONSET DATE<br>3/23/99 | 7. SOC. DATE<br>5/5/99 |
| 8. TYPE:<br>☐ PT ☐ OT ☐ SLP ☐ CR<br>☐ RT ☐ PS ☐ SN ☐ SW | 9. PRIMARY DIAGNOSIS<br>*(Pertinent medical DX)*<br>pneumonia, Parkinson's Disease | 10. TREATMENT DIAGNOSIS<br>Decrease in function 780.9 | 11. VISITS FROM SOC. |
| | 12. FREQ/DURATION (e.g. 3/Wk x 4 Wk.) | | |

**12. CURRENT PLAN UPDATE, FUNCTIONAL GOALS** *(Specify changes to goals and plan)*

| GOALS *(Short-Term)*<br>2 wks: Pt. will: 1. be Ⓘ sit→stand transfers ↔ bed, toilet, and bed-side commode. 2. Be CGA for balance after set-up in managing clothing during dressing bathing and toileting. 3. Demonstrate safe transfers and mobility with SBA from caregiver during home eval.<br><br>OUTCOME *(Long-Term)*<br>4 wks: In order to perform ADLs in her own home, pt. will be: 1. Ⓘ in mobility & transfers. 2. Ⓘ in toileting, dressing, and bathing c̄ set-up. 3. Ⓘ and safe in use of walker and w/c in facility & home. | PLAN<br><br><br>ADL retraining<br>Functional mobility<br>Safety education<br>Home Evaluation<br>Pt./Caregiver education |
|---|---|

| **I HAVE REVIEWED THIS PLAN OF TREATMENT AND RECERTIFY THIS PLAN OF TREATMENT WHILE UNDER MY CARE** | 14. RECERTIFICATION<br>FROM   6/5/99    THROUGH 6/19/99    ☐ N/A |
|---|---|
| 15. PHYSICIAN'S SIGNATURE | 16. DATE | 17. ON FILE (Print/type physician's name) |

**18. REASONS FOR CONTINUING TREATMENT THIS BILLING PERIOD** *(CLARIFY GOALS AND NECESSITY FOR CONTINUED SKILL CARE)*

Pt. has made significant progress in 2 wks. as demonstrated in her ability to sit up in bed and to sit on the side of the bed with CGA using a trapeze bar, a firmer mattress and a small bed rail. Pt. is SBA c̄ sit ↔ stand transfers ↔ bed; ambulates using walker c̄ SBA for safety ↔ bathroom. Pt. propels self in WC Ⓘ in her room but requires staff assistance to go to dining room 2° to fatigue. Demonstrates good awareness of safety precautions by using brakes during transfers. Pt. progressed from mod to min Ⓐ in dressing and bathing but requires help managing clothing, doing fasteners, and bathing back when standing due to ↓ balance and AROM. Pt. would benefit from continued ADL retraining, transfer and mobility training using assistive devices, skilled instruction and a home evaluation of mobility and safety issues at home with caregiver assistance. Rehab potential is excellent for discharge to her own apartment in daughter's home in 4 wks.

| 19. SIGNATURE *(or name of professional, including prof. designation)* | 20. DATE | 21. ☐ CONTINUE SERVICES<br>OR ☐ DC SERVICES |
|---|---|---|

**22. FUNCTIONAL LEVEL** *(at end of billing period - relate your documentation to functional outcomes and list problems still present)*

| | 23. SERVICE DATES<br>FROM                    THROUGH |
|---|---|

**Figure 11-2.** Department of Health and Human Services Health Care Financing Administration Form HCFA-701.

# Consultation

Consulting work is another area of occupational therapy practice that may use a slightly different method for documentation. Occupational therapists may consult on a wide variety of questions about which they have special expertise. For example, a psychiatric unit that relies on recreational therapists and activity aides for its activity therapy program might ask for an OT consult on a patient who has both physical and psychiatric disabilities. A newborn nursery might ask for an OT consult on a high-risk infant. An occupational therapist may be asked to evaluate a work, home, or school setting to make recommendations for safety, adaptations for work simplification, ergonomics, energy conservation, or compliance with ADA standards. An OT consultant might be used to peer review charts for quality improvement monitoring or reimbursement issues.

A consultant gives a professional assessment of what needs to be done, rather than actually doing it. Two of the most common requests for occupational therapy consultations are for consultation on individual consumers, or for consultation on the context in which the consumer works or resides.

## Individual Consumers

A consult on an individual consumer is written in the consumer's medical record, just as any OT note would be. In a POMR, the note is written in chronologic order in the progress note section, and might be done in a SOAP format. In a source oriented record, the consult would more likely be written in a different format, and would be found in the section of the record marked "Consults." It might be in the form of a letter or memo, or it might be written on some kind of form that the consulting OT uses routinely. The following note documents a consultation provided for a psychiatric patient who had positioning needs, and is written in SOAP format so that you can see how that would be done. In Chapter 13 there is an example of a consultation on an individual patient done in a different format.

# Hospital and Rehabilitation Center Psychiatric Unit
# Occupational Therapy Consultation Note

**Date:** 7/12/99            **Time:** 10:30 AM

Mr. E was seen at the request of Dr. Andrews to evaluate his positioning needs.

**S:** *Consumer reports that he is not able to find a comfortable position in his wheelchair, and that he is not able to propel it in a straight line due to a drag on one of the wheels.*

**O:** *Consumer noted to be leaning to the Ⓡ with increased pressure on the Ⓡ elbow. Back of wheelchair noted to be hammocking badly. Armrests do not provide a good position for functional use of arms. Gel cushion in chair seems to be working well as an anti-pressure device but transfers cold to consumer. Upon inspection, Ⓛ wheel found to have hairs wound around the axle, and also in need of oiling.*

**A:** *Several changes in the wheelchair are needed to increase comfort and functional use:*
*1. Add an anti-sling insert to the back of the chair to provide a more upright posture.*
*2. Add a pad to the gel cushion to prevent cold transfer of gel to consumer and also for ease of cleaning in case of incontinence.*
*3. Ⓑ arm bolsters are needed for w/c arm rests to bring consumer's arms closer to midline for ↑ functional use.*
*4. Clean and oil wheels at axle.*

> **P:**    *The adaptations listed above have been ordered. Consumer to be reevaluated after the wheelchair is repaired and adapted.*

Lisa Petty, OTR/L

## Settings in Which the Consumer Works or Resides

In evaluating a patient's home or workplace prior to discharge, a SOAP note might also be used. For an example of a home evaluation, see Chapter 13. However if a work setting were evaluated for ergonomic correctness or for ADA compliance as a whole rather than in relation to one specific patient, a letter or standardized evaluation form would be more appropriate. The following letter documents a work site evaluation that was done on a consulting basis.

# Hospital and Rehabilitation Center
# Occupational Therapy Department
## *MEMO*

**To:**    Earl R. Young, R.Ph.
**From:**  Charlet Quay, OTR/L
**Re:**    Computer ergonomics in the pharmacy
**Date:**  April 14, 1999

On the above date a visit was made to the second floor pharmacy in response to your request to perform an ergonomic evaluation of the computer workstations located there. This is in response to complaints of carpal tunnel pain, neck, and shoulder discomfort.

The following are my recommendations:

1.   **Computer keyboards** must be positioned low enough so that the shoulders can be relaxed during sustained usage and so that wrists can be maintained in neutral position rather than in extension or flexion. When the wrist is in extension or flexion there is more stress on the median nerve that is compressed in the carpal tunnel and may cause pain.

     The best position may be achieved by lowering some of the keyboards and/or angling them so the wrists can be kept neutral. Sometimes keeping the keyboards flat or even inclining them with the far end slightly down may help keep the wrists in neutral position. A wristrest used in conjunction with the keyboard is helpful to some users.

     If an ergonomic keyboard is used to avoid wrist deviations it still must be positioned so the wrists are not either flexed or extended. The correct position for each person will be slightly different since all body builds are different. It will be important for each user to know the correct body mechanics and be able to make some adjustments in the workstation to meet his/her needs.

2.   The **chair** should support the back well while maintaining the trunk in an upright position (not leaning back or forward). Thighs should be supported and the entire foot should be supported while sitting in a chair at a computer station. Foot support may be either the floor or a footrest (flat or angled) as needed to support the feet. The rungs attached to the high stools do not allow adequate foot support and may tend to disrupt back alignment. Adjustable height chairs are recommended to meet individual needs.

3.   The **monitor** needs to be placed directly in front of the viewer so it is not necessary to maintain a rotated position of the neck and trunk. Several monitors were angled to the side, requiring the user to maintain asymmetrical posture, causing neck and back strain. The height of the monitor should be adjusted so the eyes of the viewer look directly for-

ward onto the upper 1/3 of the screen. This prevents neck strain that can occur if the viewer has to look up for sustained periods of time.

4.  If the **mouse** is to be used with any frequency it should be positioned near the keyboard rather than requiring a forward reach. A wristrest attached to the mousepad is preferred to remove stress from the heel of the hand.

5.  Ideally it seems that the computer workstations should be lowered from high counters to normal table or desk work height. Table top should ideally be 26″ from floor and the distance eye to screen should be 26 to 30″. However, it is possible to manage the existing problems with the correct chairs, footrests, monitor positioning, and keyboard mouse positioning.

6.  Taking a break every 30 minutes to do some active movement and stretching exercises is recommended. A copy of sample exercises was left in the pharmacy.

If you plan to purchase chairs, footrests, etc., it would be best to actually go to an office supply vendor to try out specific pieces of furniture, or arrange to have the items on loan so the potential users can check the fit. I hope this is helpful. Please let me know if I can be of further assistance.

# Different Formats for Notes

Remember that SOAP is just a format—an organizational structure that may be used for any type of note. An initial evaluation can be written in a SOAP format, as can a treatment or progress note. There are other styles of notes that may be used instead.

**Checklists, flow sheets**, and other **similar forms** created by the facility are often used instead of SOAP notes to save time. These are an especially popular way to document an initial assessment because they allow quite a lot of information to be communicated with little time spent writing. The evaluation and discharge form presented in *Chapter 10: Documenting Different Stages of Treatment* was developed by Capitol Region Medical Center in Jefferson City, Missouri. It is a particularly good example because it covers a lot of areas in a small space without sacrificing the ability to individualize the information. It also documents the performance areas before the performance components, so that no time is wasted documenting performance components that do not impact function. Using the same form for both evaluation and discharge allows the reader to evaluate progress toward goals easily. There is ample space for comments so that the form can easily be individualized. Sometimes checklists or flow sheets are also used for treatment notes or progress notes.

**Narrative notes** are not formally organized into sections the way SOAP notes are organized. Narrative notes may present any information in any order desired. Good narrative notes usually contain the "A" data of the SOAP note. Narrative notes reporting primarily the "A" data are becoming more popular due to time and space constraints.

**DAP** notes are an adaptation of the SOAP format used in some facilities. In this format, the "D" (data) section contains both the "S" and the "O" information.

**BIRP** or **PIRP** notes are sometimes used in practice settings. Information in this format is distributed as follows:

> *B: The **behavior** exhibited by the patient*
> *I: The treatment **intervention** provided by the therapist*
> *R: The patient's **response** to the intervention provided*
> *P: The therapist's **plan** for continued treatment, based on the patient's response*
>
> *P: The **problem/purpose** of the treatment*
> *I: The **intervention** provided by the therapist*
> *R: The patient's **response** to treatment*
> *P: The **progress** and/or updated **plan***

If you work in a facility that uses one of these formats, you categorize your information slightly differently than you do when you are writing a SOAP note.

# Electronic Documentation

As we move into the 21st century, productivity standards become more stringent, and therapists' time becomes tighter, we are beginning to see more electronic documentation. This is bringing changes to the way we approach the documentation task, as well as to the format in which we write. For some, the ultimate electronic goal is a "single comprehensive, multiprovider lifelong health record" (Abdelhak, Grostick, Hanken, & Jacobs, 1996, p. 669). Before we get to this, however, there are many problems to be solved. The ease of access must be weighed against confidentiality. More tools must be developed. At present, we have a wide variety of niche products, many of which may be useful in occupational therapy practice. There are many software packages available to make our jobs easier and more efficient.

There are packages available to schedule our days as well as to send and receive mail, to evaluate our patients, to compile our treatment plans, to write our notes, and to remind us when everything is due. Software packages for electronic systems offer us a menu from which to choose the initial evaluations we want to use and to print the forms for recording the data. Other packages offer us choices of problems, goals, objectives, and possible intervention strategies rather than requiring us to compose these for individual patients. Such software can make our job simpler and save valuable health care dollars. However, there are pitfalls to be avoided in using electronic systems (Abdelhak, Grostick, Hanken, & Jacobs, 1996).

First, there is a temptation to interact solely with the computer in selecting goals, objectives, and treatment strategies, rather than including the patient in the process. This should be avoided, regardless of the extra time involved in setting goals and choosing intervention strategies **with** the patient rather than **for** her. Effective treatment requires the teamwork of the patient and therapist working toward mutually selected and agreed upon goals.

Secondly, there needs to be a way to individualize each section of the treatment plan or progress note. A good program will allow editing options or places for comments so that the documentation can be individualized to the patient. Medicare reviewers in the past have not looked favorably on "canned" plans and notes that were selected entirely from menus. One way to make an effective compromise between selecting from a menu and individualizing the statements is to use a mix-and-match system in which the menu offers components of the statement and allows the therapist to choose the components appropriate to the individual patient.

Finally, we need to make certain that the patient is our main focus, fitting the software to the patient's needs, rather than fitting the patient into the capabilities of the software package.

# CHAPTER 12
## Making Good Notes Even Better

Now that you have learned to write functional problem statements and measurable goals and objectives for effective SOAP notes, it is time to review your work and refine the skills that are not yet to the highest level of which you are capable. We will begin with problem statements and goals.

# WORKSHEET 12-1
## *Problem Statements*

As you recall, a problem list is developed from your initial assessment. Problems are then written as statements of performance areas and performance components, with a measurement device if possible.

**Consider the following problem statements. Decide whether each one is written as you have learned to write problem statements. If there is one that is not written in the best possible way, please suggest a better way to write it.**

*Pt. unable to dress LE Ⓘ due to ↓ trunk stability.*

*Pt. unable to dress self 2° Ⓡ hemiparesis.*

*Pt. unable to tolerate more than 15 minutes of functional activity due to ↓ endurance.*

# WORKSHEET 12-2

## *Goals*

You will remember that after you assess your patient, you and the patient will develop a treatment plan, containing long-term goals (discharge goals) and short-term goals (objectives). The objectives are steps to the long-term goals. You know how to write goals and objectives using the FEAST method to be sure that all the necessary components are present. However, writing the components in that order sometimes leads to a very awkward sentence.

**Try rewriting the following goals in a more logical order, making sure that conditions are present in the goal statement.**

*Pt. will pivot while standing with SBA during toilet transfers in 1 day.*

*Pt. will be min Ⓐ in dressing, UE and LE in 10 days.*

*Pt. will be min Ⓐ in toileting (dressing component) in 3 days.*

# WORKSHEET 12-3

## *SOAPing Your Note*

**Indicate beside each of the following statements under which section of the SOAP note you would place it.**

_____ Pt. supine→sit in bed Ⓘ.

_____ Pt. moved kitchen items from counter to cabinet Ⓘ using Ⓛ hand.

_____ Problems for patient are decreased coordination, strength, sensation, and proprioception in left hand.

_____ Pt. reports that his fingers are stiff this morning and that he is having trouble handling small items like buttons.

_____ Pt.'s ↑ of 15 minutes in activity tolerance for UE activities permits her to prepare a light meal Ⓘ.

_____ Pt. seen in OT clinic for evaluation of hand function.

_____ In order to return to work, pt. will demonstrate an increase of 10 lbs. grasp in Ⓛ hand by 1/3/98.

_____ Mod Ⓐ in dressing is due to patient's decreased proprioception and motor planning.

_____ Retrograde massage to Ⓡ hand and forearm with lotion performed for edema control.

_____ Pt.'s correct identification of inappropriate positioning 100% of the time would indicate memory WFL.

_____ Pt. reports that she cannot remember hip precautions.

_____ Pt. would benefit from further instruction in total hip precautions in lower body dressing, bathing, and hygiene to incorporate hip precautions into daily activities.

_____ Learning was evident by patient's ability to improve with repetition.

_____ Pt. demonstrates knowledge of her limitations in endurance by asking to take rest breaks.

_____ Pt. has progressed to a 3+ muscle grade of extension in Ⓡ wrist extensors.

_____ Pt. completed weight shifts of trunk x 10 in each of anterior, posterior, left and right lateral directions in preparation for standing to perform home management tasks.

# WORKSHEET 12-4
## *Subjective*

One common error made by new therapists in writing the subjective section of the note is that of simply listing anything important the patient had to say about his condition. All the information is relevant, but does not form a coherent whole. Again, this is not wrong, and is better than reporting irrelevant data. But it is less skillful than reporting an organized and coherent summary of what the patient had to say. Most of this patient's comments have to do with transfers.

**In the space below, write a more concise version of this "S."**

*Pt. told OT she has really bad arthritis in her right shoulder and knee.*
*Pt. told OT, "It hurts to stand on my leg." Pt. stated, "It [sliding board] needs to be moved further up on the seat."*
*When asked if she was ok after the transfer, she said, "I'm just tired."*
*Pt. stated, "I'm through," and requested help to get nearer the bed.*
*When pt. transferred to the bed, she said, "This is the hardest part."*
*Pt. stated she prefers to approach transfers from the affected side.*

## Objective

Consider the following observation of a treatment session. What does it need to make it better?

> *Pt. was seen in room for further ADL assessment. Pt. participated in ADLs and transfer activities.*
> *ADL*
> > *Pt. donned robe* Ⓘ *with set up.*
> > *Pt. donned/doffed socks* Ⓘ *with set up.*
> *MOBILITY*
> > *Bed → chair with CGA*
> > *Supine ⇆ sit* Ⓘ

This note does not have enough information. It is *too* concise. There needs to be some indication that skilled occupational therapy was provided. As it stands, it is apparent that someone observed the patient dress and transfer and recorded assist levels, but this could have been done by a rehabilitation aide or nursing staff. Secondly, the time required to do the activities documented in this note could be very short. If this is an hour treatment session, what else was done? If the patient was slow to do the things recorded above, what caused so few activities to take so long? Is there a cognitive problem? Is there a coordination, safety, or motor planning problem? Were adapted techniques or adaptive equipment used to allow the patient to be Ⓘ? Third, with this patient's documented level of independence, there is nothing in this note to justify further skilled OT. Unless this is the last session that will be provided, there needs to be information provided that will justify continued treatment.

# WORKSHEET 12-5
## *Objective*

Now it's your turn. What does this note need to make it better?

*Toilet transfers max Ⓐ*
*Toileting —* Min Ⓐ *with SBA 2° inability to support self with* Ⓛ *arm and to dress*
*UE dressing —* Min Ⓐ *, verbal cues, set up,* Ⓘ *in pulling shirt over head*
*LE dressing —* Min Ⓐ *pants to hips*
Max Ⓐ *pants to waist*
Mod Ⓘ *don* Ⓛ *shoe (elastic shoelaces)*
Mod Ⓐ *to don* Ⓡ *shoe*
*Eval of* Ⓡ *wrist, hand to assess appropriate splinting*
Ⓡ *fingers — small spasticity (index finger greatest amount)*
Ⓡ *thumb — cmc jt. painful in abd. & flex.*
Ⓡ *wrist — flaccid*

# WORKSHEET 12-6

## *Assessment*

After you have written your observation of the treatment session, you assess the meaning of the data you have put in the "O." This is the heart of your note, and shows your critical thinking skills.

**For review, write the assessment section of a SOAP note for the following patient observation.**

*Patient seen in OT clinic to work on functional movements of Ⓡ UE, dynamic sitting balance, and cognitive skills. Pt. needed mod Ⓐ in shifting weight to get to edge of w/c and max verbal cues to use correct posture and shift feet during standing pivot transfer w/c → mat. Pt. requires max verbal cues to initiate grasp of bag in beanbag activity. Pt. needs mod Ⓐ in reaching with Ⓡ UE. Pt. demonstrated ability to complete UE shoulder flexion required to toss bag appropriately 2 feet with max verbal cues. Pt. demonstrated cognitive understanding of activity with mod verbal cues by stating desired goal to be achieved by accurate aim.*

# WORKSHEET 12-7

## *Plan*

Now that you have assessed the note, write a plan for continued OT treatment.

# WORKSHEET 12-8

## Assessment and Plan

Now let's do it again. Here is your "O." Write an assessment and a plan based on this information.

*Pt. seen bedside in order to work on trunk stability, midline crossing, and bilateral integration in order to improve performance of basic ADLs.*

***Posture and balance:*** *Pt.'s posture appears slightly asymmetrical in that he laterally flexes to left and bears weight mostly on Ⓡ hip. Head turned slightly to Ⓡ; shoulders are asymmetrical; Ⓛ shoulder is elevated and protracted.*

***Vision:*** *Pt.'s visual perceptual skills appear WFL*

***Following commands and expression:*** *Pt. able to follow verbal commands 100% of the time and he displays appropriate affect during conversation 100% of the time.*

***Movement:*** *When asked to reach forward with Ⓛ UE, pt. used compensatory technique of elevating Ⓛ shoulder and laterally flexing to Ⓡ. While midline crossing to Ⓛ, pt. required verbal cues to shift weight to left and to incorporate Ⓛ UE. Pt. required muscle tapping in order to depress Ⓛ shoulder during reach patterns.*

***Transfers and dressing:*** *Pt. required max Ⓐ for trunk stability in transfer bed → w/c and needed max Ⓐ in dressing due to ↓ AROM of Ⓛ UE and poor trunk mobility.*

From Borcherding S. *Documentation Manual for Writing SOAP Notes in Occupational Therapy.* © 2000 SLACK Incorporated

# WORKSHEET 12-9

## A Note That Needs Some Therapy

**Take a look at this note and decide what it needs to make it better.**

**S:** Pt. unable to communicate due to aphasia.

**O:** Pt. was seen in the rehabilitation gym to increase functional movement in order to gain independence in ADLs.
**Cognition:** Pt. demonstrated ↓ ability to follow verbal instructions during tx. session. Pt. demonstrated ability to follow 1-step commands during treatment session 5/7 following multiple demonstrations and tactile cues 5/5 times.
**Balance:** Pt. demonstrated good static sitting balance as indicated on the Boone Balance scale but required mod Ⓐ to regain balance after reaching beyond arm's length.
**UE:** Pt. demonstrated ↓ coordination with Ⓛ UE movement. Pt. demonstrated poor motor control when reaching for objects and manipulating them. Pt.'s Ⓡ UE was observed to be flaccid. Pt. was observed repositioning Ⓡ UE when it fell off his lap. Pt. demonstrated ability to move his Ⓡ UE using the clasped hand method but was observed to wince in pain at movements beyond 90° of shoulder flexion. Pt. required max Ⓐ to support weight on Ⓡ UE while weightbearing when reaching positions.

**A:** Pt. would benefit from activities that encourage dynamic balance to facilitate Ⓘ with dressing activity. Pt. would benefit from ADL training to improve Ⓡ UE weakness and incoordination of Ⓑ UEs. Pt. would benefit from scapular mobilization of Ⓡ UE to ↑ FROM.

**P:** Pt. to be seen b.i.d. for 2 weeks to work on showering. Pt. will demonstrate ability to shower safely while standing with SBA in 2 weeks. Pt. will demonstrate ability to lather 80% of body with CGA in 1 week.

# WORKSHEET 12-10

## The "Almost" Note

This note is **almost** good enough. In fact, it seems quite good on the surface, but has major flaws in categories and clinical reasoning. This is a 78-year-old female who has had a Ⓛ CVA and has Ⓡ hemiparesis.

**What does this note need to make it better?**

**S:** Pt. reports stiffness in Ⓛ hip, but improvement from previous pain. She states a preference for transferring to her left. Pt. states that she is willing to do "whatever it takes to get out of the hospital."

**O:** Pt. seen in room for work on dressing and functional mobility

**Transfer:** Pt. SBA for standing pivot transfer bed → w/c to the left.
Pt. min Ⓐ with transfers w/c ⇆ toilet using grab bar

**Mobility:** Pt. SBA with VCs to flex trunk when rolling from supine to Ⓡ side
Pt. SBA supine → sit; minⒶ sit → stand
Pt. in Ⓘ w/c mobility

**Dressing:** Pt. Ⓘ in donning shirt
Pt. min Ⓐ with VCs to don bra while standing
Pt. Ⓘ in donning socks and shoes
Pt. min Ⓐ with walker and VC in donning underwear and pants
Pt. needs setup for dressing activities

**UE ROM:** Ⓛ UE—WFL
Ⓡ UE ↓ range in proximal shoulder flexion

**Static standing:** Pt. CGA with walker Ⓑ UE support

**Dynamic standing:** Pt. SBA with walker for balance

**A:** Deficits noted in Ⓡ UE coordination, Ⓑ UE strength, and dynamic standing balance. Pt. Ⓘ in dressing EOB, but is min Ⓐ in dressing when standing with a walker. Ⓛ UE AROM is WFL, but Ⓡ UE has deficits noted in shoulder flexion. Pt. needs SBA in bed mobility when rolling to unaffected side and min Ⓐ in sit → stand 2° ↓ UE strength. Pt. needs SBA for transfer to unaffected side in pivot transfer bed → w/c and min Ⓐ w/c ⇆ toilet. Pt. would benefit from skilled OT to continue UE strengthening and coordination exercises and to ↑ dynamic standing balance using walker, in order to ↑ Ⓘ in ADLs.

**P:** Pt. to be seen b.i.d. for 30-minute sessions to continue to work on dynamic standing balance. Pt. will require SBA in grooming activities standing sink-side with standard walker within 2 weeks.

# Conclusion

Congratulations! If you have read all the material presented in this manual and completed all the exercises, you should be able to document your patient care to the most rigorous standards. The notes that follow are intended to provide you with examples of well-written notes from a variety of treatment settings. These examples, along with the ones imbedded in the various chapters, should provide you with ideas for documenting some of the more common kinds of treatment sessions. If you work in a setting that is not represented, you are invited to contribute notes to the next edition of this manual.

Included at the end of this chapter is a two-sided page that summarizes everything you have learned about writing SOAP notes in occupational therapy. Another copy printed on thicker paper is also included so you can pull it out and carry it with you to use as a quick reference guide while you are learning to document.

# A Quick Checklist for Evaluating Your SOAP Note

Use the following summary chart as a quick reference guide to be sure that your note contains all the essential elements.

## S (Subjective)
☐ 1.  Use something significant the patient says about his treatment or condition.

## O (Objective)
☐ 1.  Begin this section with where and for what reason the patient was seen.

☐ 2.  Report what you see, either chronologically or using categories.

   3.  Remember to do the following:
☐      Deemphasize the media
☐      Specify what the part of the task the assistance was for
☐      Show skilled OT happening
☐      Leave yourself out
☐      Focus on the patient's response
☐      Avoid being judgmental

## A (Assessment)
   1.  In an evaluation note:
☐      Estimate rehab potential
☐      Make a problem list

   2.  In any note:
☐      Look at the data in your "O" sentence by sentence, asking yourself what each statement means for the patient's occupational functioning.

   3.  End the "A" with "patient would benefit from..."
☐      Justify continued skilled OT
☐      Set up the plan

   (Be sure the timelines and activities you are putting in your plan matches the skilled OT you say your patient needs.)

## P (Plan)
☐ 1.  Specify how often the patient will be seen and for how long.
☐ 2.  Tell what you will be working on during that time.
☐ 3.  End with a long-term goal or short-term goal, whichever is more appropriate for your patient and practice setting.

   Make certain function is integral to the note. Also make certain everything goes together. For example, if you talk about inability to dress in the problem list, don't switch to feeding in the goals and showering in the plan.

*If you have read the text carefully you will know what each item means. For a more complete explanation, refer to the chapter that provides information in detail. There is a brief explanation of SOAP guidelines on the back of this sheet.*

## S (Subjective)

Use something **significant** the patient says about his **treatment** or **condition**. If there is nothing significant, ask yourself whether you are using your interview skills to elicit the information about how the patient sees things.

## O (Objective)

Begin this section with where the patient was seen and for what reason. For example:

*Pt. seen beside for functional mobility.*

Report what you see, either chronologically or using categories.

Remember to do the following:

Focus on performance elements and deemphasize the media. For example:

*Pt. worked on tripod pinch using pegs.*

When giving assist levels, specify the part of the task the assistance was for. For example:

*Pt. min Ⓐ for correct hand placement during pivot transfer to toilet.*

Show skilled OT happening—make it clear that you were not just a passive observer. For example, don't just list all the assist levels and think that is enough.

Write from the patient's point of view, leaving yourself out. For example:

*Pt. evaluated—rather than therapist evaluated the pt.*

Focus on the patient's response, rather than on what you did. For example:

*Pt. able to don socks using dressing stick after demonstration.*

Avoid being judgmental. For example, say he *"...didn't complete the activity."* Don't add *"...because he was stubborn."*

## A (Assessment)

In an evaluation note:

Estimate rehab potential. For example:

*Rehab potential excellent to return home with caregiver.*

Make a problem list. For example:

*Problems include ½ AROM of Ⓛ shoulder, motor planning deficits...*

In any note:

Look at the data in your "O" sentence by sentence, asking yourself what each statement means for the patient's occupational functioning. This is your assessment of the data. For example, if in your "O" you noted that pt. falls to the left when sitting unsupported, what do you think this means he will be unable to do for himself? For example:

*Pt. unable to sit EOB unsupported to dress.*

End the "A" with "patient would benefit from..."

Justify continued skilled OT.

*Pt. would benefit from skilled instruction in energy conservation techniques as well as continued work on AROM of the UEs, strengthening, and compensatory techniques for performing IADL tasks one handed.*

Set up the plan.

(Be sure the timelines you are putting in your plan match the skilled OT you document that your patient needs.) For example, if you justify skilled OT by saying only that the pt. would benefit from skilled instruction in energy conservation techniques, then do not say that you plan to treat him twice a day for 2 weeks. Skilled instruction in energy conservation should take only one session, or at most two sessions.

## P (Plan)

Specify frequency and duration of treatment. For example:

*Pt. to be seen 1 hour daily for 2 weeks.*

Tell what type of performance areas you will be focusing treatment with the patient during that time.

*Pt. to be seen 1 hour daily for 2 weeks for instruction in Ⓘ bathing, grooming, and hygiene.*

End with a LTG or STG, whichever is more appropriate for your patient and the practice setting.

*By the end of the week, pt. will be able to don socks Ⓘ sitting EOB without losing balance.*

# CHAPTER 13
## Examples of Different Kinds of Notes

This chapter provides examples of notes from a variety of stages of treatment and from a variety of practice settings.

The notes in this section were written by students, faculty, and practicing therapists. The signatures are chosen to make the notes anonymous unless the person who wrote it wanted credit for his/her work, in which case the real name has been used.

**Initial Evaluation Report**

# Hospital and Rehabilitation Center
# Initial Evaluation Report

**Name:** Rebecca B.      **Age:** 80      **Date:** 5/3/99      **Time:** 8:30 AM
**Primary Dx:** Fx. Ⓛ hip  **Secondary Dx:** high blood pressure
**Primary Payment Source:** Medicare      **Secondary Payment Source:** supplemental insurance
**Admission Date:** 5/2/99    **Estimated Length of Stay:** 4 days   **Physician:** B. Garrett, M.D.
**Pertinent History:** Rebecca had gone upstairs to use the bathroom since there were none on the first floor. She became lightheaded, fell down the stairs and broke her hip. She was admitted for a total hip replacement yesterday. Her family lives out of town and cannot stay with her. She wants to return home.

**S:**  *Pt. stated that she would like to "get this leg well" and go home to "live a regular life." She reports living alone and being Ⓘ in all ADLs prior to admission.*

**O:**  *Pt. seen in room for initial evaluation of morning ADL capabilities after THR. Pt. educated on use of ADL equipment for self-care tasks and adherence to hip precautions. Pt. demonstrated ability to repeat 2/4 precautions. During ADL evaluation pt. was observed flexing 8° to 10° beyond 90° and required four verbal cues to remain at or below 90° during the 45-minute session. Other three hip precautions were followed Ⓘ. Pt. able to complete sponge bath at sink after set up for upper body, and used dressing stick with washcloth and verbal cues for lower body. Pt. was partial wt. bearing on Ⓛ leg; required min Ⓐ for balance with sit↔stand to bathe back peri area. Pt. able to complete upper body dressing after set up. Pt. able to don underwear and pants over hips using a dressing stick. Pt. able to don socks using sock aid after set up with verbal cues. Pt. able to complete grooming tasks and oral care Ⓘ. Following verbal cues, pt. demonstrated good problem-solving by trying different body positions to perform ADLs while adhering to hip precautions and demonstrated understanding of adaptive aids by utilizing reacher and dressing stick correctly after instruction. Pt. demonstrated ↓ ADL tolerance as she required four 2-minute rest breaks during dressing tasks. Pt. then seen in OT clinic for physical evaluation.*

   *Ⓑ UE AROM—WFL*     *Ⓑ UE strength—WFL*
   *UE sensation-intact*      *Grip strength Ⓡ47#, Ⓛ43# (Ⓡ hand dominant)*
   *Tripod pinch Ⓡ 10#, Ⓛ 1#*   *Lateral pinch Ⓡ 10#; Ⓛ 1#*

**A:**  *Pt. demonstrated good motivation, problem-solving skills, and understanding of equipment use. Upper body strength and AROM WFL, all of which indicate excellent rehab potential. Pt. is able to complete grooming tasks and oral care Ⓘ but is unsafe to complete lower body dressing and bathing due to ↓ activity tolerance, balance, and inconsistent compliance with hip precautions. Problem areas include ↓ balance in sit↔stand, ↓ ADL activity tolerance, and ↓ safety in ADL tasks. These problem areas negatively impact pt.'s ability to be Ⓘ and safe in ADL tasks. Pt. would benefit from skilled instruction on hip precautions and use of adaptive equipment with ADL performance, therapeutic activities that facilitate dynamic standing balance and ↑ ADL activity tolerance. Exploration of interim living arrangement or possible continued home visits and home equipment procurement if progress warrants discharge to home.*

P:       *Pt. to be seen b.i.d. for 1 hour the next 3 days to* ↑ Ⓘ *in self-care tasks through instruction on hip precautions and use of adaptive equipment, with tasks to* ↑ *activity tolerance, and balance activities using reaching patterns while standing.*

## Long-term Goals:
By discharge (5/7/99) pt. will:
1.     Safely complete lower body dressing and bathing modified Ⓘ utilizing adaptive equipment with 100% adherence to hip precautions.
2.     Be Ⓘ and safe in toileting using adaptive equipment of walker and bedside commode.

## Short-term Goals:
By 4th tx. session, pt. will:
1.     Demonstrate ability to don shoes & socks 100% of time Ⓘ, utilizing adapted techniques & devices with 100% adherence to hip precautions.
2.     ↑ ADL tolerance as demonstrated by no more than one 15 sec. rest break during lower body dressing task of donning slacks.
3.     Safely bathe her peri area modified Ⓘ utilizing adaptive techniques and devices with 100% adherence to hip precautions.

By next tx. session pt. will transfer with SBA sit↔stand using bedside commode and manage clothing with no more than two verbal cues.

By 2nd tx. session, pt. will be Ⓘ in sit↔stand using walker.

By 3rd tx. session, pt. will be assessed for possible continued home visits and home equipment procurement if progress warrants discharge to home.

Kim Student, OTR/L

# Treatment Plan

**Name:** Rebecca B.     **Age:** 80     **Primary Dx:** Left hip fracture/THR
**Strengths:** UE strength and AROM; intact cognition and motivation to return home

**Functional Problem:** Unsafe in ADL tasks due to ↓ compliance with hip precautions following THR, ↑ fatigue, ↓ endurance for ADL tasks requiring frequent rest breaks.

## Long-term Goals:
By discharge (5/7/99) pt. will safely complete LE dressing and bathing utilizing adaptive equipment with 100% adherence to hip precautions.

| STG (By 5/5/99 pt. will:) | Interventions |
|---|---|
| 1. Demonstrate ability to don shoes and socks 100% of time with no verbal cues, utilizing adapted techniques and devices with 100% adherence to hip precautions.<br>2. ↑ ADL tolerance as demonstrated by no more than one 15 sec. rest break during dressing task of donning slacks.<br>3. Safely bathe her peri area utilizing adaptive techniques and devices with 100% adherence to hip precautions. | 1. Instruct and have pt. verbalize 4/4 hip precautions.<br>2. Instruct in use of adaptive techniques/devices followed by demonstration of use in dressing and bathing activities.<br>3. Educate pt. & provide written instructions on energy conservation techniques. Evaluate understanding by her application during ADL tasks; ask about how she performs ADL tasks at home.<br>4. Instruct in manipulation of clothing and bathing items while standing in walker at sink s̄ violating hip precautions. |

**Functional Problem:** ↓ dynamic balance during ADL tasks.

**Long-term Goals**

By discharge (5/7/99) pt. will be Ⓘ and safe in toileting using adaptive equipment (walker and bedside commode).

| STG | Interventions |
|---|---|
| 1. Pt. Ⓘ in sit↔stand using walker in 2 tx. sessions while observing total hip precautions. | 1. Instruct pt. in safe transfer techniques; rein-force compliance with total hip precautions. |
| 2. Pt. will transfer with SBA sit↔stand using bedside commode and manage clothing with no more than 2 verbal cues by next tx. session. | 2. Provide UE strengthening through reaching and wt. bearing activities at sink and closet for grooming and dressing items and pushing up from chair and bedside commode. |
| 3. Pt. will be assessed for possible continued home visits and home equipment procure-ment if progress warrants discharge to home by 3rd tx. session. | 3. Interview pt. regarding home environment; explore and discuss interim living arrangements or possible equipment use and placement i home; discuss support services needed charge home is warranted. |

**Discharge Plan:** To assisted living facility for 3 to 4 wks. until safe in completing all ADL tasks Ⓘ at home with assistance of home health aide if warranted by progress.

## Treatment Plan: Cancer

# Hospital and Rehabilitation Center Treatment Plan

**Name:** Carol M.          **Age:** 35          **Primary Dx:** Ⓛ mastectomy 2° breast CA
**Strengths:** Prior to surgery Carol was in good physical condition and employed full time. She has some social support from her sister who lives in another state.

**Functional Problem:** Carol avoids social outings with friends due to ↓ self-esteem secondary to cosmetic alterations imposed by mastectomy procedure, which precludes her ability to return to work.

**Long-term Goal:**

Carol will ↑ social interactions and activity to six outings/month within the next month, in preparation for return to work.

| STG | Interventions |
|---|---|
| Carol will identify one support group of interest to her within 1 week in order to ↑ willingness to be out in public for work and social activities. | Educate Carol re: available support groups and peer visitation groups, their contact persons, telephone numbers, and ask her whether or not she has made contact. |
| Carol will attend one support group activity within 2 weeks in order to ↑ confidence in social and work situations. | Discuss Carol's experiences with the support groups with her. |

| STG | Interventions |
|---|---|
| Carol will initiate conversation with at least one other support member during her first visit to the group in order to ↓ negative impact of cosmetic alterations to body image.<br><br>Carol will enroll in a women's exercise program in order to ↑ activity tolerance and positive body image.<br><br>Carol will identify five assets she possesses other than physical in order to ↑ self esteem and confidence in social and work situations. | Accompany Carol into the community the first time she goes out.<br><br>Educate Carol re: area exercise groups for post mastectomy patients.<br><br>Discuss Carol's assets with her, encouraging her to think of as many as she can. |

**Functional Problem:** Carol is unable to return to work 2° 3/4 AROM, 4-/5 muscle strength, ↓ activity tolerance (fatigues after 1 hr.), and sensory changes.

**Long-term Goal:**
Carol will return to work part time by 8/8/99.

| STG | Interventions |
|---|---|
| Carol will demonstrate activity tolerance of 2 hours for work tasks within 3 weeks. | Scar massage and myofascial release to incision area along with pt. education on self-massage. |
| Carol will demonstrate ↑ of 20° in Ⓛ shoulder flexion in order to be able to reach the items she needs to work. | PROM to Ⓛ shoulder—instruct in self ranging program. Active resistive ROM to Ⓛ UE. |
| Carol will demonstrate strength of 5- in Ⓛ shoulder musculature in order to be able to complete repetitive tasks at work. | Resistive strengthening with theratubing, weights, and graded functional activities. Work simulation with patient education on energy conservation principles. |
| Carol will use correct body mechanics in seated and active work tasks in order to have pain level of < 2/10 while working. | Provide home exercise program and modify as patient progresses. Provide education on women's exercise groups. |
| Carol will observe sensory precautions in work and daily living tasks. | Educate in ergonomics and posture in order to prevent pain. Provide education on safety concerns with sensory loss. |

**Progress Note: Hand Therapy**

# Hand Therapy Clinic Progress Note

**Date:** 6/11/99          **Time:** 1:00 PM

**S:** Client reports pain @ the ulnar styloid with forearm supination. Client reports she is still unable to start her car c̄ her Ⓡ hand but can now use it to turn a doorknob.

**O:** Client seen in hand clinic for functional range of motion in Ⓡ UE. Moist heat applied to Ⓡ hand and forearm for 10 minutes prior to beginning treatment.

A/PROM Measurements for hand and forearm are:
[KEY:     flexion/extension; ( ) PROM; - extension lag; + hyperextension]

| Ⓡ hand | MP | PIP | DIP |
|---|---|---|---|
| Index | 0/90 | 0/105 | 0/75 |
| Long | 0/90 | 0/105 | 0/80 |
| Ring | 0/90 | 0/105 | 0/80 |
| Small | 0/90 | -14/105 (0/105) | 0/79 |

Ⓡ Wrist:     +45/40 composite   (+60/50) composite        +45/50 non-composite
Ⓡ forearm:  Supination 62 (78)  Pronation 90

Client performed the following exercises c̄ Ⓡ UE:
Isometric forearm supination x 10, AAROM supination x 5, AROM forearm supination x 5. After exercise, client's supination ↑ to 77° AROM. HEP revised to include blue foam for flexion strengthening 2 to 3 x day.

**A:** Client's gains in DIP flexion AROM since last week are due to ↑ strength of flexors. Active wrist extension ↑ 9° and extension ↑ 5° from last week. ↑ in active pronation is due to ↑ strength while client lost 14° of forearm supination since last week which appears to be a result of muscle tightness. Client would benefit from continued skilled OT to regain FROM to complete IADLs and for general strengthening.

**P:** Client to be seen 2 x wk. for 30-minute sessions. Continue wrist exercises and modify treatment plan to include more supination stretching and strengthening. Client will demonstrate Ⓘ in HEP and sufficient ↑ in Ⓡ forearm supination to start her car c̄ Ⓡ UE in 2 weeks.

Laurie Student, OTR/L

## Progress Note: Mental Health

# Behavioral Health Center Progress Note

Date: 5/21/99          Time: 4:00pm

S:    *During the first 3 days of admission, Ms. Jones elected not to attend OT group sessions, maintaining that she was too "anxious and overwhelmed."*

O:    *Client stayed in her room most of the time for first 3 days despite consistent invitations to attend groups. On this day the client attended a stress management group. Initially she was quiet, but gradually began entering into the activity. She was able to identify specific physical, emotional, and behavioral symptoms that she experiences when feeling overwhelmed or anxious. Ms. Jones stated that she had not been aware of these stress reactions.*

A:    *The client is making progress as indicated by her initiating attendance to group, as well as relaxing and opening up socially during the group. Additional progress indicated by recognizing specific symptoms of stress as opposed to relating only general feelings.*

P:    *Continue all goals as originally stated. Client to be seen daily to provide opportunities for Ms. Jones to learn basic stress management techniques so that she may recognize and control stress reactions when she begins feeling overwhelmed or anxious.*

David Clinician, OTR/L

## Discharge Note (SOAP format)

# Hospital and Rehabilitation Center
# Occupational Therapy Discharge Summary

Patient: Ted Davis                      Admit Date: 1/29/99
OT order received: 2/7/99               OT Evaluation completed: 2/8/99
Number of treatments: 5                 Discharge Date: 2/16/99

S:    *Pt. reports "doing a lot better" and being "less confused" than he was on admission.*

O:    *Pt. initially presented with multiple trauma 2° to MVA. OT evaluation on 2/8/99 indicated pt. had deficits in short-term memory, safety awareness, attention to task, and ADL status. Pt. seen 30 minutes daily for 5 days for ADL retraining for dressing, grooming and functional mobility. Pt. and family received skilled instruction in safety precautions in the home. Pt.'s functional status on admit and discharge as follows:*

| Goal # | Admit status | Goal | D/C status |
|---|---|---|---|
| 1 | Min Ⓐ in grooming | Set up/supervision | Set up/supervision |
| 2 | CGA in toilet transfers | SBA | SBA |
| 3 | Supine→sit with min Ⓐ | SBA | SBA |
| 4 | Min Ⓐ UE dressing | Set up/supervision | Set up/supervision |

**A:**     *All goals achieved due to improved cognitive status, awareness of safety precautions, and skilled instruction in ADLs. Pt. will need supervision at home 2° remaining cognitive (attention and short-term memory) deficits.*

**P:**     *Pt. discharged to home. Recommend home health OT evaluation for safety in home environment and potential for necessary durable medical equipment. No home exercise program given. No other referrals at time of discharge. OT will follow up in 1 month by phone to check pt.'s functional status in the home.*

Laura Student, OTR/L

## Discharge Note (Facility format)

# Hospital and Rehabilitation Center Discharge Summary

**Name:** Marjorie Patient                    **Medical Record#:** 97865
**Physician:** Fred Dietrich, MD              **Room #:** 537
**Start of Care:** 4/1/99                     **Date of Discharge:** 4/10/99
**Primary Dx:** Ⓡ CVA                         **Secondary Dx:** Arthritis

__X__ Occupational Therapy        ____ Physical Therapy        ____ Communicative Disorders

**Course of Treatment:** Client seen daily for 9 days, 30 minutes each session following CVA to work on ↑ independence in self-care skills, functional mobility, UE strengthening, energy conservation, and activity tolerance.

**Status on Discharge:** Client reports feeling much better and is ready to go home.

**Discharge Status**                         **Admit Status**
Self-care Ⓘ and safe                          Self-care mod Ⓐ
Functional mobility Ⓘ and safe                Functional mobility mod Ⓐ
Activity tolerance 8 minutes for ADL tasks    Activity tolerance 10 minutes for ADL tasks

**Goals Met:** Client has met self-care and functional mobility goals using energy conservation techniques.

**Goals Not Met:** Activity tolerance goal not met due to client refusing last two treatment sessions when she learned she was being discharged.

**Patient/Family Education:** Client instructed in and demonstrates understanding of HEP. Handouts given. Client reports having weights at home she can use for continued UE strengthening as instructed in her HEP.

**Recommendations:** Discharge client to her sister's home due to goals being met. HEP attached. No home health recommended at this time.

Bonnie Student, OTR/L

The notes that follow are meant to enlarge the scope of the treatment notes and practice settings found in this manual. These notes were chosen with an eye to their variety.

**Treatment Note: Acute Care**

# Hospital and Rehabilitation Center Acute Care Unit
# Occupational Therapy Treatment Note

**Date: 4/22/99**          **Time: 3:00 pm**

S:  *Pt. non-verbal. Pt. demonstrated startle response c̄ position change.*

O:  *Pt. seen bedside to work on initiating and attending to self-care task. When asked to point finger, pt. required multiple verbal cues and demonstrations, and demonstrated poor response time. Pt. requires max Ⓐ supine→sit EOB. Pt. required multiple verbal cues and hand over hand Ⓐ 75% of the time to initiate holding on to washcloth. Pt. able to bring washcloth to water with one verbal cue but required hand over hand Ⓐ to bring washcloth to face. Pt. attended to looking at self in mirror for ~ 1 minute. Pt. required hand over hand Ⓐ to initiate brushing hair. Shoulder AROM limited due to ↑ tone.*

A:  *Overall, pt.'s motor planning, task initiation, and attention during treatment activities continues to be limited. Pt. would benefit from ranging activities to increase shoulder elevation, as well as further interventions focusing on the skills of initiating and attending to task in order to complete ADL activities.*

P:  *Pt. to continue OT daily for 20-minute sessions until discharge in ~ 4 weeks to work on self-care activities and the underlying performance components necessary to complete tasks Ⓘ. Pt. will follow a 1 step command in 1 week in order to attend to self-care routine.*

Susan Student, OTR/L

**Treatment Note: Cognition**

# Hospital Occupational Therapy Treatment Note

**Date: 4/5/99**          **Time: 10:00 AM**

S:  *Veteran reports feeling fine, but says he does not remember the OTRs name that he has been working with.*

O:  *Veteran seen in OT clinic for cognitive tasks, Ⓡ UE AROM, strengthening, and fine motor coordination. Veteran oriented to person, month, year, and place after prompting. He followed 2 step commands after max verbal cues and mod physical assist to complete basic self-care tasks. Veteran was unable to grasp and release items with Ⓡ hand. He required mod physical and verbal cues to complete UE AROM used in table top activities.*

**A:** *Veteran is not oriented to surroundings at all times, which presents safety concerns. His ↓ cognitive functioning leads to ↓attention to completion of tasks, specifically dressing, feeding, and bathing. Veteran would benefit from cognitive skills training and safety instruction. Veteran also displays ↓ strength, coordination, and AROM in Ⓡ UE which limits his ability to complete ADL activities. He would benefit from instruction in using Ⓡ UE as an assist as well as from activities to ↑ Ⓡ UE strength, AROM, and coordination to perform self-care activities.*

**P:** *Veteran will be seen daily for 4 weeks for 1 hour to improve cognitive skills, ↑ attention to task and safety awareness, and to ↑ Ⓡ UE strength, AROM, and coordination in order to complete self-care tasks. Veteran will attend to task for 3 minutes in order to complete morning grooming within 2 weeks.*

Patty Student, OTR/L

## Consulting Note

This consulting note is not done in a SOAP format, since it is designed to be sent to the school rather than written in the child's medical record. This note also provides an example of a note that is done by a student co-signed by the supervising occupational therapist.

# Motor Skills Clinic

**Name:** Brianne Elyse Sample          **Date of Birth:** May 20, 1991
**Date of Evaluation:** July 25, 1996   **Chronological Age:** 5 years and 2 months
**Parents:** Irma and Jim Sample         **Phone:** (555) 888-3988
**Address:** 123 Lewis Street, Columbia, Missouri  65211

Brianne Elyse Sample is a 5-year, 2-month-old girl who is being seen today upon request of her family and the kindergarten program that she attends. Brianne was an active, healthy child, until April of 1996 at which time she developed Haemophilus influenzae type-B meningitis. Brianne was hospitalized for 10 days and had a "long recovery" by the family's report. Even though Mr. and Mrs. Sample feel that Brianne has now made a full recovery, they are concerned that this illness slowed her previously fast progress and that she may not be ready for kindergarten this fall. The parents and the program are requesting an evaluation to assess her readiness for kindergarten.

### Assessment Results

The Fine Motor Section of the Peabody Developmental Motor Scales (PDMS First Edition, 1983) was administered to Brianne on July 25, 1996. The PDMS is a standardized norm-referenced evaluation designed to assess fine and gross motor skills in children birth to 83 months of age. Today's evaluation of Brianne (at chronological age 5 years and 2 months) reveals:

|                        | PDMS Fine Motor Skills |      |
| ---------------------- | --------- | --- |
|                        | T-Score   | DMQ |
| Total Fine Motor Score | 56        | 109 |
| Subsections:           |           |     |
|     Grasping | 73 | 135 |
|     Hand Use | 73 | 135 |
|     Eye-Hand Coordination | 59 | 114 |
|     Manual Dexterity | 53 | 104 |

\* T-Scores are based on a mean of 50 and a standard deviation of 10.

* DMQ Scores are based on a mean of 100 and a standard deviation of 15.

Brianne was alert and cooperative throughout the 25-minute evaluation. She exhibited an evolving right hand dominance—utilizing the right upper extremity as the main initiator of activity and the left upper extremity as an assist and stabilizer. Posture, muscle tone, strength, and endurance all appeared to be within normal limits for chronological age. Response to auditory stimuli in the environment was appropriate. The parents do not report any hearing or vision concerns. During the evaluation, the child did not squint, rub eyes, nor exhibit any difficulties with visual regard/tracking.

### Summary

Results of the Fine Motor Section of the Peabody Developmental Motor Scales (given on July 25, 1996) indicate that Brianne Elyse Sample is functioning slightly above the mean in the area of fine motor skills at chronological age 5 years and 2 months. Motor coordination and response to environmental stimuli appear to be within normal limits for chronological age. Even though Brianne was recently hospitalized with a serious illness, she currently exhibits adequate fine motor abilities to perform kindergarten activities.

### Actions Taken

Evaluation results were discussed with Brianne's parents who attended the evaluation session today. A copy of this report will be sent to the family and to the kindergarten program as requested by the family.

### Plan

Reevaluation upon request.

Truman T. Tiger, OTS
_____
Date

Christy L.A. Nelson, MS, OTR/L
_____
Date

cc:   Irma and Jim Sample               Dictated: July 25, 1996
      Kindergarten program              Typed: July 27, 1996

## Treatment Note: Early Intervention

# Neonatal Follow-up
# Outpatient Clinic Occupational Therapy Note

**Name:** Bobby D.      **Age:** 11 Months      **Date:** 3/25/99      **Time:** 8:30 AM
**Primary Dx:** r/o developmental delay
**Primary Payment Source:** Blue Cross      **Secondary Payment Source:** none
**Pertinent History:** Bobby is an 11-month, 11-day old male child whose adjusted age is 9 months 27 days. He was initially discharged from hospital on August 18, 1997 (chronologic age 1-04-08; adjusted age 0-01-24). Since discharge, Bobby has been seen twice for medical evaluation at hospital (11-7-98 and 1-18-99). He is being seen today for his first OT developmental evaluation as a part of the Outpatient Neonatal Follow-up Program. His mother is present at the evaluation.

> S:      *Child is not yet old enough to use language to communicate, but makes sounds ("ba, da, ma," etc.) WFL for overall developmental level.*

O:      Today's evaluation reveals:
        a.      Atypical patterns of posture and movement (persistent primitive reflexes, presence of tonic reflexes, moderate increase in muscle tone, limited repertoire of movement, and postural asymmetry
        b.      Possible visual difficulties (immature visual tracking and intermittent mal-alignment—one/both eyes drift inward)
        c.      Delayed milestones (child exhibits skills clustering around the 4 to 6 month developmental level)

A:      These findings indicate that this child is experiencing developmental delay, deviance in the pattern of development, and possible visual difficulties. Bobby would benefit from the following plan of care.

P:      The mother has been informed of the results of the evaluation, and is in agreement with the following plan:
        a.      Occupational Therapy will contact the Neonatal Follow-up Clinic physician regarding vision concerns.
        b.      Family is scheduled to return on April 7, 1999 at 9 am to begin joint OT/PT therapy program
        c.      Plan to reevaluate developmental status in 3 months just prior to the next Neonatal Follow-up Clinic appointment.

Christy L.A. Nelson, OTR/L

## Treatment Note: Home Evaluation

# Hospital and Rehabilitation Center
# Occupational Therapy Home Evaluation Report

**Date:** 2/27/98          **Time:** 3:40 PM

S:      Pt. stated numerous times how nice it was to be home. Pt. verbalized more in this setting than at the facility.

O:      Prior to admission, pt. lived at home alone with support from family, home health nurse, and housekeeping aide and was Ⓘ with all ADLs. The following are the results of a home evaluation:
        **Entry:** 2 ½" step, 4" door jam. Uneven grass to step. Concrete broken and no railings present.
        **Kitchen:** 26" area around table in center of kitchen, 27" between snack bar and fridge, 30" high snack bar located on outskirt of kitchen. Little room to maneuver safely. Needs utensils and appliances within reach.
        **Hallway:** 22" from dining room → bedroom with bathroom between inaccessible for walker. Remainder of entries adequate to accommodate walker.
        **Bathroom:** 17" floor to tub top, 18" floor to toilet seat. Bathroom small, but can accommodate wheeled walker.
        **Other:** Throw rugs in all rooms. Chair blocks bedroom access with wheeled walker. End tables block access to living room from dining room with wheeled walker.

A:    With the following modifications and recommendations, the home would be acceptable for pt. to return to after discharge:
Remove all throw rugs to decrease falls; remove excess furniture to increase walking area and increase safety.
Adaptive equipment needed—raised toilet seat with safety rails, shower chair with back support, grab bars, and hand-held shower.
Add railing to hallway to increase safety without walker.
Add railing and repair concrete to outside entry.
Remove kitchen table and utilize snack bar or dining table to increase mobility in kitchen.
Lower telephone by back door to improve reach.

P:    Resident and family will implement the preceding recommendations and changes to allow discharge from facility to return home safely.

Carrie Student, OTR/L

## Treatment Note: Home Health Visit

# Home Health Agency Visit Note

**Date:** 2/4/99          **Time:** 8:30 AM

S:    Patient stated that he was "shaky" from his shower earlier in the AM. Pt.'s daughter reported that pt. showered and dressed with min Ⓐ for balance and coordination to manage fasteners. Pt. reported that he has been following his HEP.

O:    Pt. seen in his home to assess balance, coordination, level of compliance, and Ⓘ c̄ HEP and to introduce new hand strengthening exercises. Pt. required mod verbal cues to initiate and complete pre-existing HEP.

New hand strengthening exercises added—finger spread with rubber bands of various sizes; intrinsic muscle coordination worksheet, for example, pen rolling, etc.

Pt. and daughter participated in discussion about planning treatment activities to compliment patient's interests. Gun repair projects and small woodworking activities were suggested for coordination and strength in hands. Pt. demonstrated good static sitting balance throughout the session, but needed CGA for balance to stand safely from chair.

A:    Pt. demonstrates good understanding of HEP through participation, but required verbal cues to initiate the activity, raising continued concerns about compliance. Pt. demonstrates ↑ strength c̄ Thera-Band exercises from 1/29/99 through increased repetitions and decreased fatigue. Now handles 1" items such as pajama buttons Ⓘ but has difficulty with smaller items. Rehab potential is excellent. Pt. would benefit from continued skilled OT to further instruct in energy conservation techniques, safety, and to modify HEP as needed.

P:    Pt. to be seen 2 x wk. for 1 hour sessions to continue work on self-care Ⓘ. Pt. will demonstrate Ⓘ in showering and buttoning shirt by 3/5/99.

Stacy Student, OTR/L

**Treatment Note: Home Health Mental Health**

# Community Support Services Contact Note

**Name:** John Williams    **Date:** 2/14/99    **Beginning Time:** 9:00 AM    **Ending Time:** 10:45 AM
**Length of Service:** 75 minutes    **Goal:** 2, 4, and 5

S:    *John states that having a bank account instead of keeping all his money in cash in an envelope is very confusing to him, and he is never sure anymore how much money he has. He also reported some continuing confusion regarding his medication.*

O:    *John was seen in his home to fill his mediset and review his grocery needs. Skilled instruction provided in meal planning and calculating probable food costs. He was then taken to the bank to withdraw some money, and to a local grocery store to purchase food. At the bank, the teller figured John's account, which confused him. Skilled instruction provided in calculating a bank balance. At the grocery store, John purchased canned fruits and vegetables, ground beef, fresh lettuce, and a loaf of bread. Upon returning home he put the lettuce and meat in the refrigerator Ⓘ and consulted his weekly menu planner to determine what he had planned for lunch.*

A:    *John needed only two verbal cues to fill his mediset with correct doses of all medications this week as opposed to four verbal cues last week. Understanding a bank balance is a new skill for John and he needs continued skilled instruction and opportunities to apply his new knowledge before he is able to manage the account Ⓘ. He continues to make progress in choosing healthy foods as evidence by his Ⓘ choice of canned fruits and vegetables and the addition of lettuce to his sandwiches. John could benefit from continued skilled instruction in ADL skills such as Ⓘ management of medication, food, and money in order to be able to live Ⓘ in the community without the support of a professional staff.*

P:    *John will continue to be seen weekly in his home and community settings in order to work toward Ⓘ in meeting his daily needs. John will fill his mediset Ⓘ without verbal cues within 3 weeks in order to ↓ the amount of support needed to comply with his medication regimen.*

Alan Thomas, OTR/L

**Treatment Note: Mental Health**

# Mental Health Center Occupational Therapy Treatment Note

**Date:** 4/16/99        **Time:** 4:00 pm

S:    *Client reported she is currently not volunteering and has not worked for the past 4 years due to her disability status. Regarding volunteering, she says, "I need the structure," and further stated that she wants to be productive. Currently, client reports she sleeps "too much," and is having relationship problems.*

O: Client was admitted yesterday and attended 4/4 group sessions today. During expressive therapy group, client participated in baking with the rest of the group, but did not eat anything. When each group member identified current emotions, client identified hers as miserable, angry, very anxious, overstimulated, frustrated, frightened, and alienated. During skills group, client identified a possible problem she may encounter upon discharge to be lack of organization, with her "red flags" being oversleeping and agitation. Client welcomed suggestions from others regarding structuring her time.

A: Client is very perceptive of her emotions and limitations. Her refusal to eat with the group indicates continued appetite disturbance. Client would benefit from information about eating disorders. She would also benefit from continued group participation, with emphasis on increasing self-esteem and time management skills. Client's participation in all four group sessions today indicates good rehab potential.

P: Client will continue to attend all daily group sessions while on the acute unit to work on increasing self-esteem and ability to structure her time. Client will demonstrate increased time management skills by naming five strategies she will use for gaining control of her daily time by D/C in approximately 4 days.

Nancy Student, OTR/L

## Treatment Note: Pediatric (Preschool Age)

# Children's Center Occupational Therapy Treatment Note

Date: 4/7/99          Time: 3:00 PM

S: Mary said she wanted to play, but when the task was difficult for her, she said, "You do it. You fix it."

O: Mary seen in her home to work on Ⓑ use of UE to ↑ spontaneous use of Ⓛ hand as a functional assist, sitting balance while tailor sitting unsupported, and functional mobility, as a prerequisite to self-care and play skills. Mary was engaged during ~ 90% of the session.
*Bilateral UE Use:* Mary required max Ⓐ to pull shirt over stuffed animal's arms with Ⓡ UE while holding it with Ⓛ UE. She spontaneously used Ⓛ hand to assist with stabilizing animal while pulling sleeve over its arm and shoulder c̄ Ⓡ hand. Mary initiated snapping shirt, but needed max Ⓐ to use Ⓛ hand to stabilize shirt while fastening snaps. Ⓑ hands used to hold animal steady during play.
*Sitting Balance:* Mary requires touch cues from stand → sit in walker and mod physical Ⓐ from side sit → cross-legged sit. She demonstrated adequate sitting balance to play for 5 minutes, requiring tactile cues twice to right herself from a lateral tilt.

A: Mary demonstrated Ⓑ coordination and use of Ⓛ hand as a functional assist ~ 60% of the time, which is an increase from last week. When she is engrossed in activity, Mary is unable to concentrate on postural support, and needs CGA assist to resume upright posture. She would benefit from continued skilled OT for activities which challenge postural support in order to gain protective responses, body righting, and vestibular integration in order to ↑ her Ⓘ during play.

P:    *Mary will be seen weekly for 7 weeks to continue strengthening postural support in
      order to ↑ her Ⓘ in play activities and promote Ⓑ hand use and ↑ use of the Ⓛ
      hand as a functional assist during ADL and play activities. Mary will be able to
      maintain upright posture for 10 minutes without lateral tilt within 3 weeks.*

Julie Student, OTR/L

## Treatment Note: Public School

# Children's Center Visit Note

Date: 4/12/98                Time: 2:30 pm

S:    *Heather did not use verbal language to communicate, but did echo words spoken to her.*

O:    *Heather was seen in classroom to work on fine motor skills to prepare for scissors
      and improve prehension patterns for writing. After 5 minutes of brushing to decre-
      ase tactile sensitivity, Heather worked on palmar pinch and tripod grasp prehension
      patterns using a "Fruit Loop" bracelet activity for 20 minutes. Heather used tongs
      (in preparation for scissors use) to pull 15 Fruit Loops out of a cup one at a time.
      Then using a palmar pinch, she placed each Fruit Loop over a pipe cleaner. Five ver-
      bal cues were required for task completion.*

A:    *Heather manipulates tongs well and exhibits a good awareness of positioning of
      tongs within her hands, which is an indicator that proper scissors use will be
      attained soon. Good attention to task for entire 25 minutes.*

P:    *Continue prehension activities 3 x wk. using a variety of media in 20- to 30-minute
      intervals until proper scissors use goal is achieved. Heather will be able to cut a
      piece of 8"x10" paper ~ in half using adaptive spring scissors Ⓘ by 2/19/98.*

Durwood Student, OTR/L

## Treatment Note: Prosthetic Adaptation

# Hospital and Rehabilitation Center
# Occupational Therapy Note

Name: Daniel Patient              Date: 2/5/98    Time: 3:06 PM        Physician: Dr. Woodard
Medical Record #: 87654           Room #: 455W

S:    *Pt. appeared pleased with adaptations to prosthetic leg fasteners made this date
      stating, "This will work."*

O:    *Pt. seen in rehab gym for adaptations necessary to don/doff prosthesis. Pt. sit ⇆
      stand Ⓘ from w/c while keeping one hand on walker for support. Pt. positioned
      prosthetic leg and attempted to fasten straps. Pt. mod Ⓐ in fastening of straps, Ⓘ
      in undoing of straps to doff prosthesis. Adaptations of prosthetic leg harness com-
      pleted this date.*

A:     Inability to don prosthesis Ⓘ currently limits Ⓘ with ambulation/functional toileting. Pt. would benefit from additional skilled instruction in use of pulley-like fasteners on prosthesis to allow one-handed closure installed this date.

P:     Pt. will don/doff prosthesis Ⓘ with added pulley system using strap/loop/velcro by end of next tx. session. Will continue to see pt. daily for 2 more days.

Joanie Student, OTR/L

## Treatment Note: Safety

# Hospital and Rehabilitation Center
# Occupational Therapy Treatment Note

**Date: 4/22/99          Time:     10:15 AM**

S:     Pt. reports ↓ activity tolerance and ↑ shortness of breath with exertion. Pt. reports feeling OK about asking nursing for Ⓐ c̄ dressing, but has urgent incontinence and cannot always wait for Ⓐ to manage $O_2$ cord to toilet.

O:     Pt. seen in room to assess safety during toileting.
**Cognition:** WFL; no deficits
**Functional Mobility:** Pt. uses walker, his difficulty managing $O_2$ cord, requires SBA for safety.
**Upper Extremity Strength:** WNL; Pt. fatigues c̄ use of UE.
**ADL:** Pt. CGA for clothing management c̄ toileting. Mobility during toileting and dressing requires min Ⓐ for $O_2$ cord management and safety. Pt. dresses with mod Ⓐ due to ↓ activity tolerance, and needs to stop p̄ 5 minutes dressing activity.

A:     Pt. at risk for falls due to inability to manage $O_2$ cord during functional mobility to toilet. Pt. would benefit from adaptive equipment and techniques to toilet with ↑ Ⓘ as well as instruction in energy conservation techniques and ↑ activity tolerance for ADL tasks.

P:     Pt. will be seen 2 x wk. for 1 week in order to ↑ Ⓘ and safety in toileting. Pt. will be able to use toilet safely and Ⓘ in 1 wk.

Paige Student, OTR/L

## Treatment Note: Splint

# Hospital and Treatment Center Outpatient Clinic
# Occupational Therapy Note

**Date: 1/21/99          Time: 3:00 PM**

S:     Mr. J. stated that the pain in his right wrist and thumb was "not as bad as it was 2 weeks ago." He reported that his splint is rubbing a calcium deposit on the dorsum of his hand and that he is not wearing the splint at work during the day. He also reported feeling pain during treatment with movement of the Ⓡ thumb, and that ice and iontopheresis ↓ pain.

O:     *Mr. J. arrived at OP clinic wearing forearm based thumb spica splint. Upon removal of splint, wrist appeared slightly swollen.*
*AROM*

| | |
|---|---|
| *wrist flexion ~25%* | *wrist extension < 25%* |
| *thumb flexion and extension ~25%* | |

*Mr. J. tolerated ~3 minutes friction massage over abductor pollicis longus and extensor pollicis brevis tendons. Ice applied for 5 minutes; Mr. J. instructed in using ice at home and at work to ↓ pain by ↓ inflammation of tendons. Splint reformed to eliminate rubbing on dorsum of hand, and Mr. J. instructed in wearing schedule at work. HEP modified and Mr. J. demonstrated new procedures correctly.*

A:     *Swelling ↓ since last tx. session. Wrist and thumb AROM are ~ 50% below functional limits, due to pain upon movement. Limited AROM & pain are causing functional problems in the work environment. Ice and iontopheresis ↓ pain and therefore ↑ functional ability $\bar{c}$ ® hand. Splint reconstruction will also contribute to ↓ pain. Mr. J. would benefit from continued skilled OT to ↓ pain, ↑ AROM, ↑ ability to use ® hand at work.*

P:     *Continue to see Mr. J. 2 x wk. for the following:*
*Ice & iontopheresis to ↓ pain in ® hand and wrist.*
*Friction massage to ↓ inflammation and ↑ AROM in ® wrist and thumb.*
*Reevaluation of splint for fit and use after reconstruction.*
*Reevaluation of effectiveness and compliance of HEP.*
*To achieve goal of ↓ pain in ® wrist and hand for use in functional activity at work and home, pt. will use a screwdriver during work task with <3/10 on pain scale within 2 visits (1 wk.).*

Laura Student, OTR/L

## Treatment Note: Wheelchair Evaluation

# Hospital and Rehabilitation Center
# Occupational Therapy Note

**Date:** 2/5/99        **Time:** 1:00 pm

S:     *Client states, "I could get out more with a power wheelchair, like to the shopping center." Client c/o fatigue when ambulating and states that he is not able to drive anymore.*

O:     *Client seen in OT clinic for power w/c evaluation. Current manual w/c is narrow, causing sides of client's hips to press arm rests into wheels making propulsion difficult. Consult $\bar{c}$ PT reveals client fatigues and has muscle spasms when ambulating distances of > 100 ft. Client measured for power w/c.*
*22" wide*
*18" seat depth, 17" knee to floor*
*18" seat to mid-scapula*

*w/c features discussed with DME representative. 60° and 90° footrests tried on manual w/c; client prefers 90° rests for comfort. Joystick control to be placed on Ⓡ armrest due to Ⓛ 2° hemiparesis. Client requests full armrests to accommodate positioning Ⓛ UE and greater support in transitioning sit → stand. Client able to answer questions regarding powered mobility and accessibility in the home and community, and to problem-solve for transportation needs such as OATS bus, local accessibility points and terrains, and using manual w/c for family visits.*

A:     *Client has reasonable expectations and understanding for accessibility, mobility, and transportation issues. Potential for using powered w/c is excellent. Client would benefit from skilled instruction in driving w/c using joystick control.*

P:     *Client to be seen b.i.d. for 2 days prior to d/c home to work on w/c positioning, adjustment, and driving safely. Client will maneuver powered w/c safely in indoor/outdoor settings by d/c on 2/9/99.*

Desiree Student, OTR/L

# BIBLIOGRAPHY

Abdelhak, M., Grostick, S., Hanken, M. A., & Jacobs, E. (Eds.). (1996). *Health information: Management of a strategic resource.* Philadelphia, PA: W. B. Saunders.

American Council for Occupational Therapy Education. (1998a). *Standards for an accredited educational program for the occupational therapist.* Bethesda, MD: Author.

American Council for Occupational Therapy Education. (1998b). *Standards for an accredited educational program for the occupational therapy assistant.* Bethesda, MD: Author.

American Occupational Therapy Association. (1998a). Elements of clinical documentation (Revision). In *The reference manual of the official documents of the American Occupational Therapy Association, Inc.* (pp. 141-150). Bethesda, MD: Author.

American Occupational Therapy Association. (1998b). Service delivery in occupational therapy. In *The reference manual of the official documents of the American Occupational Therapy Association, Inc.* (pp. 99-104). Bethesda, MD: Author.

American Occupational Therapy Association. (1998c). Standards of practice for occupational therapy. In *The reference manual of the official documents of the American Occupational Therapy Association, Inc.* (pp. 317-323). Bethesda, MD: Author.

American Occupational Therapy Association. (1998d). Uniform Terminology for occupational therapy—third edition. In *The reference manual of the official documents of the American Occupational Therapy Association, Inc.* (pp. 155-168). Bethesda, MD: Author.

American Occupational Therapy Association Managed Care Project Team. (1996). *Managed care: An occupational therapy sourcebook.* Bethesda, MD: American Occupational Therapy Association.

Cullen, C. (1998). *Medicare documentation for occupational therapy* [On-line]. Available: http://www.geocities.com/Heartland/Prairie/5309/physdis.html

Huffman, E. K. (1994). *Health information management.* Berwyn, IL: Physician's Record.

Kannenberg, K. (1998). Special consideration III: Mental health. In J. D. Acquaviva (Ed.), *Effective documentation for occupational therapy* (pp. 115-129). Bethesda, MD: American Occupational Therapy Association.

Lopes, M. (1998). *Medicare guidelines explained for occupational therapy service delivery.* (T. J. Slominski, Ed.). Gaylord, MI: Northern Speech Services.

Moyers, P. A. (1999). *The guide to occupational therapy practice.* Bethesda, MD: American Occupational Therapy Association.

O'Hara, D. J. (1990). *Guidelines for writing a S. O. A. P. note.* Unpublished manuscript, University of Missouri-Columbia.

Pedretti, L. W. (1996). *Occupational therapy: Practice skills for physical dysfunction.* St. Louis, MO: Mosby.

Ramsey, R. M., & Auerbach, E. (1997). Forms follow function: Documentation for reimbursement in mental health OT. *OT Practice, 2,* 20-23.

# BIBLIOGRAPHY

# APPENDIX
## Suggestions for Completing the Worksheets

The worksheets in this manual were originally developed for use as in-class exercises. In a classroom situation, students are asked to collaborate on an answer and their collaborative efforts recorded on a flip chart or blackboard. This is a particularly non-threatening way for students to learn new skills, since it allows them to try out ideas and hear the ideas of others as they work toward a correct result. In this situation the instructor can guide their efforts by asking questions to facilitate good clinical reasoning.

In my experience, many of these exercises do not work as well when used as homework assignments. Because there are so many "correct" ways to complete them, they can be grading nightmares. The suggestions offered here as "good" or "correct" are only a few of the many possible correct answers. As you do the exercises with a class, you may collect many more equally "good" answers.

If you are a new therapist or student using this manual, rather than an instructor, you should be able to work your way through the exercises and check your work against those in this Appendix. Remember that your answer can be different and still be correct, as long as it contains the essential elements. You should not sacrifice your own writing style to be more like someone else's, as long as your information and protocol are essentially correct.

SOAP notes are very difficult to write if there is no treatment session about which to write. Although there are many examples in this manual, there is no substitute for observing or working with actual patients. Only then will you be able to translate your treatment session onto paper in a meaningful way.

# Chapter 2

## Worksheet 2-1: Using Abbreviations

Translate each sentence written with abbreviations into full English phrases or sentences.

Pt. c/o pain in ⓇMCP joint p̄ ~ 15 min. PROM.
> *Patient complained of pain in the right metacarpophalangeal joint after approximately 15 minutes of passive range of motion.*

Pt. w/c → mat c̄ sliding board max Ⓐ x 2.
> *Patient transferred from his wheelchair to the mat using a sliding board and maximum assistance of two people.*

Pt. O x 4.
> *The patient was oriented to person, time, place, and situation.*

Pt. able to don pants SBA c̄ verbal cues to thread Ⓛ LE.
> *The patient was able to put on his pants with stand-by assistance, but needed verbal cues to be able to thread his left foot into the leg hole.*

1° dx. THR 2° dx. COPD & CHF.
> *Primary diagnosis is total hip replacement. Secondary diagnoses are chronic obstructive pulmonary disease and congestive heart failure.*

**Shorten these notes using only the standard abbreviations in your syllabus.**

Patient has thirty degrees of passive range of motion in the left distal interphalangeal joint which is within functional limits.

*30° PROM in Ⓛ DIP is WFL.*

Patient is able to put on her socks with standby assistance, but requires moderate assistance with putting on and taking off left shoe.

*Pt. dons socks SBA but requires mod Ⓐ to don & doff Ⓛ shoe.*

The patient requires contact guard assistance for balance during her morning dressing which she performs while sitting on the edge of her bed.

*CGA for balance for AM dressing EOB.*

## Worksheet 2-2: Additional Practice
**Shorten these notes using only the standard abbreviations in your syllabus.**

The patient was seen bedside for training in activities of daily living. She was able to perform bed mobility exercises with moderate assistance, but needed maximum assistance to put on her Depends. She was able to go from a supine position to a sitting position with minimum assistance and from a sitting position to a standing position with moderate assistance.

*Pt. seen bedside for ADL training. Mod for Ⓐ bed mobility, max Ⓐ to don Depends. Supine → sit min. Ⓐ and sit → stand mod Ⓐ.*

The resident came to the occupational therapy clinic via wheelchair escort. The resident was observed to lean to his left. The resident needed verbal cues and minimum assistance in positioning his body in the wheelchair to maintain midline orientation and symmetrical posture. The resident transferred from his wheelchair to the toilet with moderate assistance of one person using a standing pivot transfer. He needed verbal cues and visual feedback from a mirror to maintain upright posture.

*Resident to OT via w/c escort. Resident leans Ⓛ and needs verbal cues and min. physical assist to maintain symmetrical posture in midline. Standing pivot transfer w/c → toilet mod Ⓐ. Verbal cues and feedback using a mirror needed to maintain upright posture.*

The veteran was seen in his own room seated in a wheelchair for an initial evaluation. The veteran's short-term memory was three out of three for immediate recall, one out of three after 1 minute, and zero out of three with verbal cues after 5 minutes. The left upper extremity shoulder flexion was a grade of 4, shoulder extension was a grade of 4, elbow flexion was a grade of 4, elbow extension was a grade of 4, wrist extension was a grade of 4 minus, wrist flexion was a grade of 4 minus, and grip strength was at 8 pounds. The left upper extremity muscle grades are within functional limits and the left upper extremity light touch is intact.

*Veteran seen in room seated in w/c for initial eval. Short-term memory 3/3 immediate recall, 1/3 after 1 minute, 0/5 c̄ verbal cues after 5 min. Ⓛ shoulder and elbow strength grade 4, wrist strength 4-, grip strength 8# all WFL. Light touch intact.*

# Chapter 3

## Worksheet 3-3: Writing Functional Problem Statements

Without having seen the patient in question, it is impossible to know exactly what the correct problem statement would have been. Here are some possible ways that functional problem statements might have been written for the problems given:

1.     The client has acquired an injury to his brain. As a result, he is not able to pay attention to task for very long at a time, and is having trouble completing his morning routine. Usually he can pay attention to what he is doing for about 2 minutes, and needs to be redirected back to the task after that.
   *< 3 minute attention span 2° ABI interferes ability to complete ADL tasks.*
   *Pt. needs min verbal cues to complete dressing due to attention span of < 3 minutes.*
   *Pt. able to attend to dressing activity for ~2 minutes 2° ABI.*

2.     The resident is not very cognitively aware. She has trouble figuring out what to do first if she has to complete a complex task, and she doesn't remember what she has just been told.
   *Pt. needs max. verbal assistance in toileting due to ↓ ability to sequence steps of task.*
   *Pt. requires >5 verbal cues to brush teeth due to ↓ short-term memory.*
   *Memory and sequencing problems result in safety concerns.*
   *Inability to sequence 3 step task interferes c̄ ability to carry out IADL tasks.*

3.     Mr. J. has recently sustained a Ⓡ CVA. His Ⓛ upper extremity is flaccid and he forgets it is there.
   *Pt. requires mod Ⓐ to dress upper body due to flaccid Ⓛ UE and Ⓛ side neglect.*
   *Pt. max. Ⓐ donning shirt over UE due to Ⓛ side neglect as a result of Ⓡ CVA.*
   *Pt. mod Ⓐ in feeding due to flaccidity in dominant Ⓛ UE.*
   *Flaccidity in Ⓛ UE and Ⓛ neglect results in mod Ⓐ in grooming and hygiene.*

4.     The patient is unable to transfer w/c ⇆ toilet by himself. One of the primary reasons he cannot transfer is because he must observe total hip precautions. In addition, there are strength and balance problems.
   *Pt. requires max Ⓐ w/c ⇆ toilet due to unstable dynamic sitting balance.*
   *Pt. requires mod Ⓐ to transfer w/c ⇆ toilet due to ↓ UE strength.*
   *Pt. mod Ⓐ transfer w/c ⇆ toilet due to hip precautions 2° recent THR.*

5.     The veteran has increased tone in his formerly dominant Ⓡ upper extremity. He is referred to OT to work on ADL tasks.
   *Pt. mod Ⓐ in UE dressing due to severe spasticity.*
   *Moderate spasticity in Ⓡ UE results in illegible handwriting.*
   *Pt. unable to grasp eating utensils due to mod. spasticity of Ⓡ UE.*
   *Pt. mod Ⓐ in over-the-head method of donning shirt due to spasticity of Ⓡ shoulder adductors and internal rotators.*
   *Pt. unable to don shirt 2° high tone in Ⓡ UE.*

# Chapter 4

## Worksheet 4-1: Choosing Goals for Medical Necessity

**What other problems might this woman have due to decreased strength in her Ⓡ hand?**
   *Pt. unable to handle small items needed for grooming due to 2+ strength in Ⓡ UE.*
   *Pt. unable to write > 3 minutes due to 2+ strength in her Ⓡ UE.*
   *Pt. unable to fasten clothing due to 2+ strength in Ⓡ UE.*

**What LTG might you use that would show medical necessity for increasing Ⓡ UE strength?**
   *Pt. will be able to complete grooming activities Ⓘ within 1 month.*
   *Pt. will write for 15 minutes one rest break within 1 month.*
   *Pt. will be able to fasten clothing within 3 weeks.*

**What short-term goal might be used as a step to that LTG?**

*Pt. will be able to remove lid from toothpaste within 2 weeks.*
*Pt. will be able to sign first name within 1 week.*
*Pt. will be able to button one 1" button within 1 week.*

## Worksheet 4-2: Evaluating Goal Statements

Which of the following goals have each of the necessary components to be useful in occupational therapy documentation? For each goal that you find to be incomplete or inaccurate in some way, please indicate what it lacks.

1.   By the time of discharge in 2 weeks, patient will be able to dress himself with min Ⓐ for balance using a sock aid and reacher while sitting in a wheelchair.
*This goal has all the necessary components to be useful.*

2.   Patient will tolerate 10 minutes of treatment daily.
*This goal lacks a function and a time frame. In addition, the behavior (tolerating treatment) is not useful, because it is not something a patient needs to do after discharge. This would be better stated as "tolerate 10 minutes of grooming/hygiene activity."*

3.   Patient will demonstrate increased coping skills in order to live at home with her granddaughter within 2 weeks.
*This goal lacks specificity, and it needs a condition—"coping skills" is far too broad. The coping skills in question need to be specified.*

4.   Patient will demonstrate 15 minutes of activity tolerance without rest breaks using Ⓑ UE in order to complete ADL tasks before breakfast each morning.
*This goal lacks a time frame, and needs to be turned around to put function first. Patient will be able to complete basic ADL in < 15 minutes without rest breaks before breakfast each morning within 2 weeks.*

5.   In order to be able to toilet Ⓘ self after discharge, patient will demonstrate ability to perform a sliding board transfer w/c ⇆ mat within the next week.
*This goal has all the necessary components to be useful, but would be even better if the assist level of the transfer were noted ("i.e., sliding board transfer w/c ⇆ Ⓘ.")*

6.   OT will teach lower body dressing using a reacher, dressing stick and sock aid within 3 tx. sessions.
*This goal lacks a proper actor and behavior.*

7.   In order to return to living independently, pt. will demonstrate ability to balance his checkbook.
*This goal lacks a time frame, and would be even better if the assist level for balancing his checkbook were specified (i.e., "ability to balance his checkbook Ⓘ.")*

## Worksheet 4-3: Writing Realistic, Functional Measurable Goals

Without knowing the patient, it is impossible to know what the goal would really be. Here are some suggestions.

1.    **Increase attention span**
      *Pt. will attend to a cooking activity > 10 minute attention span without having to be redirected within 3 treatment sessions.*
      *Pt. will attend to brushing teeth for > 3 minutes < 3 verbal cues by 4/8/99.*

2.    **Teach the patient to follow directions**
      *In order to increase safety in IADLs within 3 weeks, patient will be able to complete a 3-step task without having to have one or more steps repeated.*
      *By the time of discharge in 2 days, patient will complete 3-step written directions for cooking a packaged meal c̄ min. assist.*

3.    **Pt. to dress upper body**
      *Pt. will be able to don shirt Ⓘ using the over-the-head method and a button hook within 2 tx. sessions.*
      *After skilled instruction, pt. will be able to dress upper body Ⓘ using one handed techniques and adaptive equipment by 9/15/99.*

4.    **Increase endurance**
      *Pt. will perform > 10 minutes of continuous standing activity in order to be able bathe her baby by discharge in 1 week.*
      *Within 2 weeks, pt. will complete 30 minutes of seated activity without rest breaks in order to return to her job as a receptionist.*
      *In order to perform light housekeeping tasks, pt. will demonstrate > 5 minutes of activity tolerance without rest breaks by discharge on 10/31/99.*

5.    **Improve money management skills**
      *Pt. will demonstrate ability to make change Ⓘ from $1.00 correctly 3/3 tries within 2 weeks.*
      *Pt. will be able to select ads from the newspaper for an apartment that rents for less than 1/3 of his regular monthly income within the next month.*

6.    **Decrease depression**
      *Pt. will spontaneously attend at least three scheduled activities per day by 4/11/99.*
      *Pt. will verbalize an interest in at least one future activity within the next 2 days.*

# Chapter 5

## Being More Coherent (page 41)

   Pt. remarked, "I can't fell anything with my hands."
   Pt. stated, "I'm wobbly as all get out today."
   Pt. expressed dizziness after bending down to touch the floor while in a seated position.
   Pt. acknowledged improvement in his sitting balance in comparison to the previous week.
While the quotations above are a very objective way of reporting the data and all the statements are relative to the treatment session, the same data could have been reported in a more concise and coherent manner, such as the following:
   Pt. expressed lack of sensation in both hands and dizziness in sitting position with dynamic movement ("wobbly" sensation). He also acknowledged improvement in sitting balance since last week.

- OR -

Pt. acknowledged improved sitting balance compared to previous week. However, he expressed dizziness after bending down while sitting and reported feeling "wobbly". Pt. also reported inability to feel anything with his hands.

## Worksheet 5-1: Choosing a Subjective Statement

In choosing what to put in your Subjective category, consider the following:

1.    *Even though the patient may have been cooperative, and even though it may have been important in this treatment session, it is an assessment of the situation, and does not belong in the "S" category of the note. The patient's social conversation might be important in some situations. However, there is a better choice for this particular note.*

2.    *In this instance, a pending visit by the patient's grandson is not really relevant to the treatment session or to how the patient sees her progress. It might be important in another situation. For example, if the patient were planning to go to live with her grandson after discharge, it might be very relevant, and might be a topic the therapist wanted to explore further with the patient.*

3.    *Feeling "pretty good" today might be important, because it might show progress or a change in her condition. In this case, however, it is not the best choice.*

4.    *The patient's observations about her upper extremity seems most pertinent to this treatment session. Use of the Ⓡ UE is relevant in all aspects of this treatment session.*

5.    *A report of safety concerns by nursing might be relevant to this patient's treatment. However, it is not the best choice for the "S" category of this note, for several reasons. A concern by nursing staff should be documented in the nursing notes. The occupational therapist should report what she sees, rather than what some other staff member believes. Finally, the subjective section of the SOAP note is used to document the atient's views about treatment rather than the staff's views, except in rare instances.*

# Chapter 6

## Worksheet 6-1: Being More Concise

**Reword the following note to be more concise.**

O:    Pt. seen bedside. Pt. ambulated ~36 inches to shower with SBA. Pt. instructed to complete shower while sitting. Pt. performed shower with SBA 2° IV line. Pt. able to wash upper and lower body Ⓘ and dry entire body after completing shower. Pt. required ~20 minutes to complete shower. Pt. then ambulated ~36 inches to chair and sat. Pt. needed verbal cues to remain seated while donning underwear and pants. Pt. able to dress UE Ⓘ and lower body with verbal cues for sitting. Pt. demonstrated good sitting balance, but needed SBA for standing. Following shower, pt. stated he would like to take a nap and was assisted back into bed.

*Pt. seen in room for self-care activities. Ambulated ~3 ft. to and from shower c̄ SBA to manage IV line while ambulating and showering. Shower took ~20 minutes. Pt. showered and dressed c̄ verbal cues to sit. Pt. demonstrated good sitting balance but required SBA for balance while standing. Following shower, pt. assisted back into bed.*

**- OR -**

*Pt. seen in room for showering and dressing. Skilled instruction provided for safety. Pt. ambulated ~3' SBA for balance. After verbal cues to sit, pt. showered in 20 min. c̄ SBA to manage IV lines. Dressed UE Ⓘ while seated and LE c̄ verbal cues to remain seated.*

## Worksheet 6-2: Being Specific About Assist Levels

Without having seen the treatment session, it is impossible to know what part of the tasks required assistance. Here are some suggestions for how the statement might have been worded:

1.    **Pt. supine → sit with min Ⓐ, bed → w/c with mod Ⓐ .**
      *Pt. supine → sit with min Ⓐ , bed → w/c with mod Ⓐ for balance.*
      *Pt. supine → sit with min Ⓐ , bed → w/c with mod Ⓐ to lift body weight.*

*Pt. supine → sit with min (A), bed → w/c with mod (A) to bring body to 45°.*
*Pt. supine → sit with min (A) swinging legs to EOB, bed → w/c with mod (A) for postural control.*

2.     **Pt. required SBA in transferring w/c ⇆ toilet**
*Pt. required SBA in transferring w/c ⇆ toilet for proper hand placement.*
*Pt. required SBA in transferring w/c ⇆ toilet to push up with arms from wheelchair.*
*Pt. required SBA in transferring w/c ⇆ toilet to remind him of steps of the transfer.*

3.     **Pt. retrieved garments from low drawers with min (A).**
*Pt. retrieved garments from low drawers with min (A) to open drawers.*
*Pt. retrieved garments from low drawers with min (A) to release trigger on reacher.*
*Pt. retrieved garments from low drawers with min (A) to judge halo placement in space.*
*Pt. retrieved garments from low drawers with min (A) to grasp handles of drawers.*

4.     **Brushing hair required max (A).**
*Brushing hair required max (A) to reach back of head.*
*Brushing hair required max (A) to flex shoulder past 35°.*

5.     **Pt. completed dressing, toileting, and hygiene with min (A).**
*Pt. completed dressing, toileting, and hygiene with min (A) to reach feet.*
*Pt. completed dressing, toileting, and hygiene with min (A) for activities requiring fine motor dexterity.*
*Pt. completed dressing, toileting, and hygiene with min (A) to adhere to hip precautions.*

# Worksheet 6-3: Deemphasizing the Treatment Media

Rewrite the following statements to emphasize the skilled OT that is actually occurring in the treatment session.

1.     **Patient played pegboard game to work on functional grasp.**
*Patient worked on functional grasp/release patterns needed to handle small objects used in grooming and dressing.*

2.     **Patient played catch using bilateral UEs to facilitate grasp and release pattern.**
*Pt. worked on functional grasp/release patterns needed to manipulate household objects.*

3.     **Patient put dirt into pot to ½ way point, added seedling, and filled remainder of pot with dirt transferred by cup. Pt. completed 3 more pots while standing 8 minutes before requiring a 5-minute rest. Pt. resumed standing position to water completed pots for approximately 5 minutes.**
*Pt. demonstrated standing tolerance of 13 minutes with a 5 minute break after 8 minutes in order to prepare for standing to complete ADL tasks.*

The treatment media also needs to be deemphasized in writing goal statements. Rewrite these two goal statements to focus on the performance area and performance components rather than on the media.

1.     **Patient will place 8 ½ inch screws and washers on a block of wood with holes while sitting by 4/10/98.**
*Pt. will demonstrate ability to handle small objects needed to return to work by placing 8 ½ inch bolts into a block of wood in < 5 minutes by 4/10/99.*

2.      **Pt. will make a clock using the appropriate materials while sitting by discharge.**
        *Pt. will demonstrate the ability to grasp, place and release objects of varying sizes needed for
        IADLs by discharge on 9/3/98.*

                                        - OR -

        *Pt. will demonstrate ability to follow written instructions by discharge on 9/3/98.*

# Chapter 7

## Worksheet 7-1: Justifying Skilled Occupational Therapy

**Which of the following meet the criterion for skilled occupational therapy?**

| | |
|---|---|
| *yes* | *Evaluation of a patient* |
| *no* | *The practice of coordination and self-care skills on a daily basis* |
| *yes* | *Establishing measurable, behavioral, objective, and individualized goals* |
| *yes* | *Developing treatment plans which are designed to meet the established goals* |
| *no* | *Carrying out a maintenance program* |
| *yes* | *Analyzing and modifying functional tasks/activities through the provision of adaptive equipment or techniques* |
| *yes* | *Determining that the modified task is safe and effective* |
| *yes* | *Carrying a breathing retraining program into ADL training* |
| *yes* | *Providing individualized instruction to the patient, family, or caregiver* |
| *yes* | *Reevaluating the patient's status* |
| *yes* | *Modifying the treatment plan based on the reevaluation* |
| *yes* | *Provision of specialized instruction to eliminate limitations in a functional activity* |
| *yes* | *Developing a home program and instructing caregivers* |
| *yes* | *Making changes in the environment* |
| *yes* | *Teaching compensatory skills* |
| *no* | *Gait training* |
| *yes* | *Intervening with patients to eliminate safety hazards* |
| *no* | *Presenting information handouts (such as energy conservation) without having the patient perform the activity* |
| *no* | *Routine exercise and strengthening programs* |
| *yes* | *Preparing a problem list which identifies present status and potential capabilities* |
| *yes* | *Adding teaching lower body dressing to a current program* |
| *yes* | *Teaching adaptive techniques such as one-handed shoe tying* |

# Chapter 8

## Worksheet 8-1: A Treatment Session Devoted to ADL Activities

Here are suggestions for the "A" and "P" sections of the note:

A:      *Resident 0 X 4 and able to make his needs known. Resident able to follow directions
if multiple means of communication used. ↓ activity tolerance limits resident's ability
to complete ADL tasks. Inability to maintain static postural control creates safety concerns in all ADL tasks. Resident would benefit from NDT to increase stability and postural control as well as continued work on ADL tasks and functional mobility.*

P:      *Resident to be seen 30 minutes b.i.d. for 14 days. Resident will complete ADL tasks
of dressing, hygiene, grooming c̄ min Ⓐ sitting EOB in 2 weeks.*

Kristen Todd, OTR/L

# Chapter 9

## Worksheet 9-1: Treatment Plan for Donald G.

The interventions used would depend on Donald's interests, the specific tasks he must perform at
work, the equipment and supplies available in the practice setting, and the skills of the therapist.
For example, if you are not qualified to do some of the physical agent modalities listed, you would
not use them. If you have had advanced practice training in Myofascial Release, you might use
that. The way these interventions are used is also important. Some might be harmful if used too
aggressively in the early stages of treatment, but would be very useful later. The following activities have been suggested for Donald:

STG: Patient will demonstrate ability to perform work-related tasks for 2 hours with a
reported pain level of < 3/10 in Ⓡ UE within 1 month.
*Physical agent modalities including:*
*Fluidotherapy Ⓡ hand and forearm*
*Iontophoresis*
*Ultrasound scar area*
*Paraffin bath*
*Heat packs*
*Massage or Myofascial Release to scar area to break up adhesions*
*Tendon gliding exercises in HEP*
*Pt. education regarding signs of use that lead to pain*
*Teach energy conservation techniques*
*Ergonomic instruction*

**STG: Pt. will demonstrate an ↑ in muscle strength of 3/5 for ℝ wrist flexion and extension with a pain level of < 3/10 within 2 weeks in order to perform work tasks.**

*Physical agent modalities preceding treatment: Moist heat, Iontophoresis*
*Worksite analysis and modification*
*Patient education based on worksite analysis*
*Use computer and mouse with correct body mechanics*
*Cooking activity using chopping, stirring, reaching*
*Spray and wash windows using arm and hand in multiple positions*
*Do laundry using washer, dryer, folding emphasizing correct body mechanics to avoid exacerbation of the problem*
*Wash dishes in warm water and put away*
*ROM arch with wrist weights*
*Home exercise program to include:*
> *Wall pushups and dowel rod exercises*
> *Thera-Band exercises*

**STG: Patient will ↑ 2# in ℝ tripod pinch strength with pain level of < 5/10 in order to perform work tasks within 2 weeks.**

*Writing activities using correct ergonomic approach*
*Use work-related items/activities that require pinching activity*
*Pick small items out of putty*
*Play games with small or weighted pieces*
*Use clothespins to hang laundry or as an exercise*
*Organize fishing tackle*
*Pick up small household objects*
*Make a pie, using pinch to arrange dough in place*
*Choose a craft activity, such as beading or leather-lacing*
*Tendon gliding exercises*
*Use nuts and bolts*

**STG: Pt. will demonstrate an ↑ of 3# in ℝ grip strength with a pain level of < 5/10 within 2 weeks in order to grasp items needed for job.**

*Simulate worksite activities graded with weights*
*Patient education based on worksite analysis*
*Videotape someone else doing the patient's job and use in patient education*
*BTE work simulator*
*Knead bread dough or play with clay with children*
*Provide compensatory strategies, such as built up handles*
*Ceramics*
*Use a pitcher to fill glasses*
*Wash the car with a large sponge*
*Polish shoes*
*Home program consisting of:*
> *Hand Helper with graded rubber bands*
> *Putty*
> *Balls and other objects to squeeze*
> *Wringing out dishcloths*
> *Tendon gliding exercises*

## Worksheet 9-2: Treatment Plan for Ginny H.

Now it is your turn. Use the following evaluation to develop a treatment plan. First, develop a problem list. Then establish long-term goals and break these down into short-term goals or objectives. Select intervention strategies that seem useful in reaching your goals and decide how often and for how long you will want to see this client. Combine all of these elements into a treatment plan.

**Name:** Ginny H.        **Age:** 87        **Sex:** F        **Physician:** B. Garrett, M.D.
**Diagnosis:** Ⓛ subdural hematoma on 4/22/99, hx. of hypertension, hearing loss
**Date of Onset:** 4/22/99        **Date of Referral:** 5/2/99        **Date of Evaluation:** 5/3/99
**Referral Source:** Nursing on 5/2/99
**History:** Prior to her stroke Ginny had been living for the last 10 years with her unmarried daughter, Sue, who is 60-years-old, and works full-time. They live in a two-story house with a bathroom on the second floor. Ginny was in acute care and has just been discharged to a rehabilitation program. She expresses a desire to return to her daughter's home. Her daughter has concerns about being able to care for her mother at home. Ginny has Medicare insurance only.

S:    Pt. expressed frustration when having difficulty brushing teeth. Pt. c/o back pain 2/10 when grooming. Pt.'s daughter said that pt. was Ⓘ in self-care prior to her stroke but has not cooked or done housework for years; further stated pt. has a hearing loss but no hearing aids.

O:    Pt. seen in room for initial assessment.
**Dressing/Grooming:** Pt. stood with CGA for 5 min while brushing teeth after setup and 2 verbal cues. Pt. Ⓘ in donning/doffing socks with extra time. Pt. continued to attempt to don Ⓡ sock using the same techniques for several minutes before being successful. Pt. did not attempt an alternative technique. Pt. mod Ⓐ in donning/doffing gown and robe due to difficulty pulling the robe around her back and threading the Ⓡ UE into the sleeve. Pt. required four 30-second rest breaks during dressing activity due to fatigue.
**Transfers/ambulation:** Pt. sit→ stand with SBA and mod Ⓐ for transfer ⇆ bedside commode due to ↓ standing balance when managing clothing. Pt. walked 3 ft. w/c → sink with CGA using walker.
**UE ROM and Strength:** All UE AROM was WNL except for Ⓑ shoulder abduction and flexion which were WFL. Ⓑ UE strength 5/5 overall except 3/5 in shoulder flexion and abduction.
**Lateral pinch (lb.):** Ⓡ 7.5; Ⓛ 9. **Tripod pinch (lb.):** Ⓡ 4; Ⓛ 7.
**Grip (lb.):** Ⓡ 29; Ⓛ 37.
**Sensation:** Light touch and sharp/dull tests indicated intact sensation Ⓑ. Pt. correctly identified 1/4 objects in the Ⓡ stereognosis test.
**Coordination:** 9 hole peg test: Placing pegs Ⓡ 52; Ⓛ 37. Removal Ⓡ 26; Ⓛ 14

A:    Self-care deficits noted in dressing and grooming 2° to ↓ activity tolerance and standing balance, weakness in Ⓑ shoulder flexion/abduction and problem-solving skills. ↓ standing balance impairs ability to transfer and ambulate Ⓘ and safely. Weakness noted in Ⓡ grasp and lateral/tripod pinch and ↓ coordination affecting fine motor coordination tasks. These problem areas negatively impact pt.'s ability to be Ⓘ and safe in ADL tasks. Rehab potential is good for returning home with caregiver assistance. Pt. would benefit from treatment to increase activity tolerance, dynamic standing balance, and safety for ADL tasks.

P:       Pt to be seen b.i.d. for 45 min. for 3 wks. to ↑ Ⓘ in self-care activities through instruction and use of adaptive equipment/techniques; to ↑ activity tolerance, standing balance and Ⓘ in transfers for functional mobility and to ↑ Ⓡ hand strength in order to be able to dress and toilet self Ⓘ . By end of 1 wk. pt. will be able to transfer safely and Ⓘ bed to bedside commode and manage clothing with SBA at walker s̄ losing balance.

**Long-term Goals:** In 3 wks pt. will be:
1.       Ⓘ in dressing and grooming.
2.       Ⓘ and safe in toileting using walker and bedside commode.
**Short-term Goals:** In 1 wk. pt. will:
1.       Demonstrate ability to don/doff gown and robe with minⒶ for set-up and verbal cues.
2.       ↑ ADL tolerance as demonstrated by ability to tolerate > 10 min. of activity first while sitting, then standing with one 30 sec. rest break.
3.       Transfer safely ⇆ bedside commode with SBA to manage clothing with no more than 2 verbal cues.
4.       In 2 wks. pt. will be assessed for possible home visit and home equipment needs.

Gayla Student, OTR/L

*Treatment Plan*
*Name: Ginny H.*        *Age: 87*        *Gender: Female*        *Date of Initial Evaluation: 5/3/99*
*Primary Diagnosis:* Ⓛ *subdural hematoma 4/22/99*        *Secondary: hx. of hypertension, hearing loss*
*Referral: Dr. Mangone*
*Frequency and Duration of Treatment: b.i.d. x 3 wks.*
*Strengths:* Ⓘ *in self-care prior to CVA; able to ambulate c̄ walker, intact sensation except for* Ⓡ *hand stereognosis; all UE AROM WNL or WFL*
*Functional Problems:*
*1.       ↓ ability to perform self-care tasks due to impaired problem-solving, ↓ coordination, ↓ stereognosis, ↓ standing balance*
*2.       safety concerns due to fatigue during ADL tasks and ↓ dynamic balance during clothing management and transfers when toileting*

| LTGs | STGs (Objectives) | Interventions |
|---|---|---|
| By discharge (5/22/99) pt. will be Ⓘ in dressing and grooming. | By 5/10/99 pt. will: 1. Demonstrate ability to don/doff gown and robe with min Ⓐ for setup and verbal cues. | Instruct pt. on upper body dressing techniques and have pt. demonstrate over-the-head and button-up methods, first in sitting and progress to standing. |
|  | 2. ↑ ADL tolerance as demonstrated by ability to tolerate >10 min. of activity while sitting or standing with one 30 sec. rest break. | Provide tactile cues to use alternative techniques; have pt. problem solve for next step of dressing or grooming tasks in sequence using visual then verbal cues as needed. Ask pt. what to do next or why this is not working now. |
|  |  | Engage pt. in reaching activities that provide a graded challenge to balance. |

| LTGs | STGs (Objectives) | Interventions |
|---|---|---|
| | 3. Be assessed for possible home visit and home equipment needs in 2 weeks. | Engage pt. in activities that ↑ AROM and fine-motor tasks such as buttoning and zipping that are graded for level of difficulty in coordination.<br><br>Educate pt. on identifying signs of fatigue. Plan rest breaks as needed to ↓ fatigue.<br><br>Perform table top activities including self-care tasks with time increasing as tolerated.<br><br>Perform deep breathing exercises and instruct in energy conservation techniques. |
| By discharge (6/22/99) pt. will be ① and safe in toileting using adaptive equipment (walker and 3-in-1 commode). | 4. Transfer safely ⇄ 3-in-1 commode when toileting with SBA to manage clothing and no more than two verbal cues in 1 week. | Instruct pt. in safe transfer techniques; reinforce compliance when transferring ⇄ bed, armchairs, 3-in-1 commode, and mat for therapeutic activities, strengthen exercises, toileting or dressing activities.<br><br>Provide ® UE strengthening and AROM through reaching and wt. bearing activities such as: reaching at sink for grooming and dressing items in graded challenging positions; pushing up from armchair and bedside commode; and table top activities of interest that require alternating support on one arm while actively reaching with the other.<br><br>Interview pt. and daughter regarding home environment; explore and discuss equipment use and placement in home; discuss support services needed if discharge to home is warranted. Schedule a home visit for assessment of pt.'s ability to manage in home environment. |

*Discharge Plan:* To home if environmental adaptations and support of caregiver and/or services are available. If pt. is not Ⓘ in self-care activities by 6/22/99, the recommendation would be to discharge to an assisted living facility for 2 to 3 wks until self-care goals are met.

Gayla Student, OTR/L

# Chapter 10
## Worksheet 10-1: Initial Evaluation Report

### Background Data
Adapted from *Elements of Clinical Documentation* (Revision) (AOTA, 1998a)

| Criteria | Compliance |
|---|---|
| Is the basic demographic data (name, age, sex, date of onset, date of admission, date of referral) present? Note any not present. | *All present* |
| Who referred the patient to OT, on what date, and what services were requested? | *Dr. Grantham for evaluation and treatment* |
| Is the patient's history and prior level of function included? | *Yes* |
| Are there any secondary problems, pre-existing conditions, contraindications, or precautions that will impact therapy? | *Diabetes* |
| What life stage or environmental factors will impact treatment? | *At 68, she would probably be retired* |
| Is the current level of function assessed? | *Yes* |
| What do the consumer and her family expect or want from treatment? | *Consumer wants to return home; family expectations not recorded* |

### Results of the Assessment

| | |
|---|---|
| What tests were used? Were there any deviations from the standard procedures? | *MME for cognition* <br> *Manual muscle test* |
| Was any other information collected besides that from the tests? | *Observation of bathing, dressing, toileting, balance, functional mobility.* |
| Are the impairments and their severity identified? | *Yes* |
| Are the functional limitations stated in objective and measurable terms? | *Problem #1–Yes* <br> *Problem #2–Yes* |
| Is the rehab potential noted? | *Yes, for modified Ⓘ in ADL activities* |

Adapted from *Elements of Clinical Documentation* (Revision) (AOTA, 1998a)

## Treatment Plan

| Criteria | Compliance |
|---|---|
| How well do the long-term goals meet the standards you have been taught? | *Functional and measurable; meet the standards* |
| Are the long-term goals reasonable in relation to the consumer's current status, rehabilitation status, and prior level of functioning? | *Yes, with only 2 weeks tx. anticipated, priorities have been set. Rehab potential is noted as good for ADLs, but if cognition does not improve it is difficult to tell whether this pt. will be able to return home despite prior level of functioning* |
| What documentation is there that the patient and family agree with the goals? | *None* |
| Do the short-term goals (objectives) relate to the long-term goals? | *Yes* |
| How well do the objectives meet the standards you have been taught? | *Functional, measurable, and action oriented; meet the standards* |
| Are the interventions that have been selected appropriate to meet the goals? | *Yes, but sketchy. More interventions would be good* |
| What assistive devices are to be used? | *Long shoehorn, schedule, list of emergency numbers* |
| What is the number, frequency, and duration of treatment? | *45 min. sessions, 5 x wk. for 2 weeks* |
| Are there any recommendations or referrals? | *No* |

Adapted from *Elements of Clinical Documentation* (Revision) (AOTA, 1998a)

## Worksheet 10-2: Treatment, Visit, or Contact Notes

| Criteria | Compliance |
| --- | --- |
| What evidence is there of the patient's participation in occupational therapy treatment? | *Detailed chronologic report of the entire treatment session* |
| What activities, techniques, or modalities were used in this treatment session? | *Washed face*<br>*Functional mobility supine → sit*<br>*Activity tolerance* |
| If any assistive or adaptive devices were used, is there documentation of whether these were fabricated, sold, or rented, its effectiveness, and what the instructions were for its use? | *None noted* |
| How did this patient (consumer) respond to the treatment provided? | $O_2$ *levels dropped and planned treatment not completed* |

Adapted from *Elements of Clinical Documentation* (Revision) (AOTA, 1998a)

## Worksheet 10-3: Progress Notes

| Criteria | Compliance |
| --- | --- |
| What treatment interventions were used? | *Assertion group*<br>*Communication group*<br>*ADL group* |
| What change has occurred in this consumer? | *Spontaneous actions*<br>*Willingness to share verbally*<br>*Unprompted attendance*<br>*Improved dress, hygiene, and makeup* |
| What goals have been continued, what goals have been changed, and what goals have been discontinued? | *Goals #1 and 2 met*<br>*Goal #3 continued*<br>*Goal #4 discontinued* |
| Have there been any changes in the time frames for reaching goals? | *None noted. Original time frame for goal #3 is unknown from this note* |
| If any assistive devices are being used, how effective are these? | *None noted* |
| What contact or conferences have there been with others? | *One would assume the social worker has been contacted about the leisure plan, but this is not explicitly noted* |
| Is there is a home program, or instructions given to caregivers? | *Leisure plan to be discussed with husband* |

| Criteria | Compliance |
|---|---|
| If there is a home program, is it attached, and is there documentation of the consumer's ability to follow it? | *No* |
| Is there a specific plan for the future? | *Only the plan for leisure time use* |

Adapted from *Elements of Clinical Documentation* (Revision) (AOTA, 1998a)

## Worksheet 10-4: Reevaluation Report

| Criteria | Compliance |
|---|---|
| What tests were readministered and what were the results? | *Manual muscle test*<br>*Grip strength*<br>*Palmar and lateral pinch strength*<br>*Results documented in note* |
| How do the current findings compare to the previous results? | *Improvement noted* |
| What are the changes in anticipated functional outcomes? | *Anticipate ① in ADL's with pt. able to return home to live with spouse* |
| What revisions are being made in the goals, objectives, and interventions? | *Goal of min Ⓐ in ADL changed to ① in ADL* |
| What revisions are being made in the frequency and duration of treatment? | *One additional week requested* |

Adapted from *Elements of Clinical Documentation* (Revision) (AOTA, 1998a)

Notice that it is possible for this note to meet the requirements and still not be a good note. This note has some excellent qualities, because it reports progress very objectively and makes the need for 1 additional week of treatment clear.

However, upon closer scrutiny, you will notice that this note has a very basic flaw. There is no beginning assessment of function, which is a critical aspect of an OT note. We know that function (bathroom safety, tub transfers) is being addressed in treatment, but we do not have a baseline against which to measure improvement. Much attention has been devoted to performance components and very little to performance areas, making it sound too much like a PT note.

## Worksheet 10-5: Discharge Summary #1 (SOAP Format)

| Criteria | Compliance |
|---|---|
| What interventions were used? | ADL retraining<br>AROM and strength |
| How many treatment sessions were there? | 15 of the 20 planned |
| How did the consumer respond? | Progress noted |
| To what degree were the short- and long-term functional goals achieved? | Partially. This is clearly noted for each activity in the discharge summary |
| How does functional status prior to therapy compare to status at discharge? | Clearly noted in the chart |
| Is there evidence that a home program was or was not given? Is it attached? | No HEP noted |
| What is schedule and specific plan for follow-up? | Plan to see under Medicare B for continued OT |
| What are the recommendations pertaining to the consumer's future needs? | Same as above |

Adapted from *Elements of Clinical Documentation* (Revision) (AOTA, 1998a)

## Worksheet 10-6: Discharge Summary #2 (Facility Form)

| Criteria | Compliance |
|---|---|
| What interventions were used? | Adaptive techniques for functional mobility, grooming, hygiene, feeding, dressing, toileting |
| How many treatment sessions were there? | 20 |
| How did the consumer respond? | Met all goals |
| To what degree were the short- and long-term functional goals achieved? | All met |
| How does functional status prior to therapy compare to status at discharge? | Status at discharge is improved |
| Is there evidence that a home program was or was not given? Is it attached? | HEP given and pt. able to perform correctly; not noted as attached |
| What is schedule and specific plan for follow-up? | PT only |
| What are the recommendations pertaining to the consumer's future needs? | Adaptive equipment recommended; continue HEP |

Adapted from *Elements of Clinical Documentation* (Revision) (AOTA, 1998a)

# Chapter 12

## Worksheet 12-1: Problem Statements

Consider the following problem statements. Decide whether each one is written as you have learned to write problem statements. If there is one that is not written in the best possible way, please suggest a better way to write it.

Pt. unable to dress Ⓘ LE due to ↓ trunk stability.
> *This problem statement would be better if the performance component were measurable, or if the problem with the performance area (dressing) were more specific.*
>
> *Pt. mod Ⓐ in dressing Ⓑ lower body due to ↓ trunk stability.*
> *Pt. mod Ⓐ to pull pants over hips due to trunk instability.*

Pt. unable to dress self 2° Ⓡ hemiparesis.
> *This problem statement would be better if the performance component was more specific, or if the performance area was more specific.*
>
> *Pt. max. Ⓐ to dress self due to ½ AROM and 3/5 strength of the Ⓡ UE.*
> *Pt. mod Ⓐ pulling shirt over head due to Ⓡ UE 3+ strength and ½ AROM in Ⓡ UE.*

Pt. unable to tolerate more than 15 minutes of functional activity due to ↓ endurance.
> *This problem statement would be better if the functional activity in question was specified, and if the amount of endurance was noted. Activity tolerance is now the preferred term for endurance.*
>
> *Pt. unable to complete morning dressing and grooming routine due to < 15 minutes activity tolerance.*
> *Pt. unable to prepare a meal due to < 5 minutes of activity tolerance.*

## Worksheet 12-2: Goals

Try rewriting the following goals in a more logical order, making sure that conditions are present in the goal statement.

Pt. will pivot while standing with SBA during toilet transfers in 1 day.
> *This goal needs a slight rewording for clarity.*
>
> *Pt. will be able to perform standing pivot transfer to toilet with SBA within 1 day.*

Pt. will be min Ⓐ in dressing, UE and LE in 10 days.
> *This goal is written in terms of what the patient will be, rather than in terms of what the patient needs. It is a small item that shows more respect to word the goal statement so that it acknowledges that the patient is more than his ability to dress himself. It also lacks the conditions under which the patient will dress himself, and specifies that he will dress only his extremities rather than his upper and lower body.*
>
> *Pt. will be able to dress self sitting EOB with min Ⓐ to pull pants over hips in 10 days.*
> -OR -
> *Within 10 days, pt. will dress self with min Ⓐ using a dressing stick and long shoehorn.*
> -OR -
> *Pt. will dress self with min Ⓐ for balance within 10 days observing 100% of hip precautions.*

Pt. will be min Ⓐ in toileting (dressing component) in 3 days.

*This goal would be better if the dressing component were integrated into the main body of the goal, and if it were clearer what the assistance was for.*

*Within 3 days, pt. will be able to pull up underpants after toileting with min Ⓐ for balance.*
-OR -
*Within 3 days, pt. will be able to manage clothing after toileting with min Ⓐ to pull pants over hips.*
-OR -
*Pt. will be able to don/doff pants after toileting with min Ⓐ to reach Ⓡ side within 3 days.*

## Worksheet 12-3: SOAPing Your Note

**Indicate beside each of the following statements under which section of the SOAP note you would place it.**

__O__      Pt. supine → sit in bed Ⓘ.

__O__      Pt. moved kitchen items from counter to cabinet Ⓘ using Ⓛ hand.

__A__      Problems for patient are decreased coordination, strength, sensation, and proprioception in left hand.

__S__      Pt. reports that his fingers are stiff this morning and that he is having trouble handling small items like buttons.

__A__      Pt.'s ↑ of 15 minutes in activity tolerance for UE activities permits her to prepare a light meal Ⓘ.

__O__      Patient seen in OT clinic for evaluation of hand function.

__P__      In order to return to work, pt. will demonstrate an increase of 10 lbs. grasp in Ⓛ hand by 1/3/98.

__A__      Mod Ⓐ in dressing is due to patient's decreased proprioception and motor planning.

__O__      Retrograde massage to Ⓡ hand and forearm with lotion performed for edema control.

__A__      Patient's correct identification of inappropriate positioning 100% of the time would indicate memory WFL.

__S__      Patient reports that she cannot remember hip precautions.

__A__      Pt. would benefit from further instruction in total hip precautions in lower body dressing, bathing, and hygiene to incorporate hip precautions into daily activities.

__A__      Learning was evident by patient's ability to improve with repetition.

__A__      Pt. demonstrates knowledge of her limitations in activity tolerance by asking to take rest breaks.

__A__      Pt. has progressed to a 3+ muscle grade of extension in Ⓡ wrist extensors.

__O__      Pt. completed weight shifts of trunk x 10 in each of anterior, posterior, left and right lateral directions in preparation for standing to perform home management tasks.

## Worksheet 12-4: Subjective

**In the space below, write a more concise version of this "S."**

Pt. told OT she has really bad arthritis in her right shoulder and knee.
Pt. told OT, "It hurts to stand on my leg." Pt. stated, "It [sliding board] needs to be moved further up on the seat."
When asked if she was ok after the transfer, she said, "I'm just tired."
Pt. stated, "I'm through," and requested help to get nearer the bed.
When pt. transferred to the bed, she said, "This is the hardest part."
Pt. stated she prefers to approach the transfers from the affected side.

> *Pt. reports arthritis in* Ⓡ *shoulder and knee, pain on weight bearing. During the transfer, pt. requested specific adjustments such as sliding board placement, proximity to bed, and approaching transfers from the affected side. Fatigue reported following transfer.*
> **-OR -**
> *Pt. reports significant arthritis in shoulder and knee and prefers to approach transfers from affected side. Pt. reports, "It hurts to bear weight on my leg." Pt. also stated w/c → bed sliding board transfers are the most difficult, and reported fatigue after transfer.*
> **-OR -**
> *Pt. reports arthritis in* Ⓡ *shoulder and knee and pain bearing weight on* Ⓡ *LE. Pt. able to verbalize needs regarding transfer (placement of board and approach from the affected side). Pt. reports fatigue after transfer.*

## Worksheet 12-5: Objective

**What does this note need to make it better?**

Toilet transfers max Ⓐ
Toileting —      Min Ⓐ with SBA 2° inability to support self with Ⓛ arm and to dress
UE dressing —  Min Ⓐ , verbal cues, set up, Ⓘ in pulling shirt over head
LE dressing —  Min Ⓐ pants to hips
                      Max Ⓐ pants to waist
                      Modified Ⓘ don Ⓛ shoe (elastic shoelaces)
                      Mod Ⓐ to don Ⓡ shoe
Eval. of Ⓡ wrist, hand to assess appropriate splinting
          Ⓡ fingers — small spasticity (index finger greatest amount)
          Ⓡ thumb — cmc jt. painful in abd. & flex.
          Ⓡ wrist — flaccid

> *First, an opening line is needed stating where and for what the patient was seen. One possibility is:*
> *Pt. seen in room for skilled instruction in ADL.*
>
> *Another possibility is:*
> *Patient seen in room for morning ADLs and splinting evaluation.*
>
> *Secondly, the categories could be reduced to three—toileting, dressing, and splinting evaluation.*
>
> *Third, it would be helpful to know why the assistance was necessary. And fourth, the UE and LE wording should be changed to upper body and lower body because the patient is not dressing only the extremities.*

***Toileting:*** *Transfers max* (A) *for balance. Min* (A) *to support self with* (L) *UE; max* (A) *to pull pants up when done.*

***Dressing:*** *Pt. able to dress upper body after setup with min* (A) *for balance when reaching further than arm's length. Pt.* (I) *in pulling shirt over head. Pt. able to pull pants up to hips with min* (A) *for balance, but needs max* (A) *to get pants up to waist using only one hand. Elastic shoelaces allow* (I) *in donning* (R) *shoe, but pt. needs mod* (A) *to get flaccid foot into* (R) *shoe.*

***Splinting Evaluation:***
  (R) *wrist: flaccid*
  (R) *fingers: min. spasticity noted*
  (R) *thumb: painful abduction and flexion at the CMC joint*

# Worksheet 12-6: Assessment

**For review, write the Assessment section of a SOAP note for the following patient observation.**

Patient seen in OT clinic to work on functional movements of (R) UE, dynamic sitting balance, and cognitive skills. Pt. needed mod (A) in shifting weight to get to edge of w/c and max verbal cues to use correct posture and shift feet during standing pivot transfer w/c → mat. Pt. requires max verbal cues to initiate grasp of bag in beanbag activity. Pt. needs mod (A) in reaching with (R) UE. Pt. demonstrated ability to complete UE shoulder flexion required to toss bag appropriately 2 feet with max verbal cues. Pt. demonstrated cognitive understanding of activity with mod verbal cues by stating desired goal to be achieved by accurate aim.

Without having seen the treatment session, it is much harder to assess the situation. Here are several possible assessments for this note:

**A:**     *Problems include deficits in motor planning, movement initiation, cognition, and muscle weakness in* (R) *UE. Activity tolerance has improved since last week from < 1 minute to > 5 minutes without a rest break. Pt. would benefit from skilled OT to increase balance, functional mobility, and grasp/release activities with involved UE in order to ↑* (I) *in self-care activities.*

-OR -

**A:**     *Decreased functional use of the* (R) *UE, decreased sitting balance, and difficulty with sequencing and problem-solving limit ability to perform ADLs. Increased shoulder flexion and motor planning since 12/15/98 and increased understanding of treatment activities would indicate good rehab potential. Pt. would benefit from continued skilled OT to increase functional AROM, exercises in grasp, exercises in weight shifting to improve dynamic sitting balance, and evaluation of both cognitive status and ability to initiate activity in order to increase* (I) *in ADL tasks.*

# Worksheet 12-7: Plan

**For review, write the Plan section of a SOAP note for the following patient observation.**

Patient seen in OT clinic to work on functional movements of (R) UE, dynamic sitting balance, and cognitive skills. Pt. needed mod (A) in shifting weight to get to edge of w/c and max verbal cues to use correct posture and shift feet during standing pivot transfer w/c → mat. Pt. requires max verbal cues to initiate grasp of bag in bean-bag activity. Pt. needs mod (A) in reaching with (R) UE. Pt. demonstrated ability to complete (R) UE shoulder flexion required to toss bag appropriately 2 feet with max verbal cues.

Pt. demonstrated cognitive understanding of activity with mod verbal cues by stating desired goal to be achieved by accurate aim.

Without having seen the treatment session, it is much harder to assess the situation. Here are two possible plans for this note:

**P:** *Pt. to be seen b.i.d. for ½ hour sessions to work on ⓡ UE movement and cognitive retraining in order to complete grooming activities with min Ⓐ. Pt. will be able to brush teeth with minⒶ by the end of fifth tx. session.*

**P:** *Continue b.i.d. for 30-minute sessions for 2 weeks to increase dynamic sitting balance in preparation for ADL training. Pt. will be able to reach for grooming items placed slightly beyond arm's reach without losing balance 3/4 times within 2 weeks.*

## Worksheet 12-8: Assessment and Plan

**Now let's do it again. Here is your "O." Write an assessment and a plan based on this information.**

Pt. seen bedside in order to work on trunk stability, midline crossing, and bilateral integration in order to improve performance of basic ADLs.
**Posture and balance:** Pt.'s posture appears slightly asymmetrical in that he laterally flexes to left and bears weight mostly on ⓡ hip. Head turned slightly to ⓡ; shoulders are asymmetrical; Ⓛ shoulder is elevated and protracted.
**Vision:** Pt.'s visual perceptual skills appear WFL
**Following commands and expression:** Pt. able to follow verbal commands 100% of the time and he displays appropriate affect during conversation 100% of the time.
**Movement:** When asked to reach forward with Ⓛ UE, pt. used compensatory technique of elevating Ⓛ shoulder and laterally flexing to ⓡ. While midline crossing to Ⓛ pt. required verbal cues to shift weight to left and to incorporate UE. Pt. required muscle tapping in order to depress Ⓛ shoulder during reach patterns.
**Transfers and dressing:** Pt. required max Ⓐ for trunk stability in transfer bed → w/c and needed max Ⓐ in dressing due to ↓ AROM of Ⓛ UE and poor trunk mobility.

**A:** *Pt.'s level of cooperation during treatment, ability to appropriately utilize visual/ perceptual skills, and ability to follow verbal commands indicate good rehab potential. Pt.'s reduced AROM of Ⓛ UE and asymmetrical trunk posture currently limit Ⓘ and safe performance of transfers and ADL tasks. Pt. would benefit from skilled instruction of bilateral integration techniques in order to incorporate Ⓛ UE in self-care activities, as well as Ⓑ UE exercises to strengthen and ↑ tone of Ⓛ UE in order to perform transfers and ADLs Ⓘ. Pt. would also benefit from skilled instruction in weight shifting techniques in order to improve trunk stability.*

**P:** *Pt. to be seen b.i.d. for 1 week in order to ↑ trunk stability, improve weight shifts, ↑ AROM of Ⓛ UE, and improve safety of transfers and ADLs. Pt. will demonstrate Ⓘ in ADL tasks by discharge on 1/7/99.*

-OR -

**A:** *Pt.'s intact cognitive status and ability to follow verbal commands indicate good rehab potential. Problems include decreased AROM and strength inⓁ UE and unstable trunk balance which limit Ⓘ in ADLs. Pt. would benefit from skilled OT to provide activities that increase AROM and strength in the Ⓛ UE, Brunnstrom balance exercises, and skilled instruction in safe transfers and dressing.*

P:      Pt. to be seen b.i.d. for 1 week for Brunnstrom balance exercises in order to begin transfer training by 1/30/99.

-OR -

A:      Safety concerns with balance noted due to asymmetry of pt.'s trunk and shoulders. ↓ AROM of Ⓛ UE and difficulty with midline crossing interferes with ability to complete ADLs. Pt.'s ability to follow verbal commands indicates good rehab potential. Pt. would benefit from AROM and strengthening activities to improve posture, balance, and trunk stability. Pt. would also benefit from future midline crossing and Ⓑ activities to prepare for future ADL training.

P:      Pt. to be seen b.i.d. for 30 minute sessions for 3 weeks for skilled instruction in AROM and strengthening exercises to ↑ trunk stability, balance, and posture. Pt. will demonstrate symmetrical posture in hips and shoulders within 2 weeks in order to sit EOB Ⓘ in preparation for ADL training.

## Worksheet 12-9: A Note That Needs Therapy

**Take a look at this note and decide what it needs to make it better.**

S:      Pt. unable to communicate due to aphasia.

O:      Pt. was seen in the rehabilitation gym to increase functional movement in order to gain independence in ADLs.
**Cognition:** Pt. demonstrated ↓ ability to follow verbal instructions during tx. session. Pt. demonstrated ability to follow 1-step commands during treatment session 5/7 following multiple demonstrations and tactile cues 5/5 times.
**Balance:** Pt. demonstrated good static sitting balance as indicated on the Boone Balance scale but required mod Ⓐ to regain balance after reaching beyond arm's length.
**UE:** Pt. demonstrated ↓ coordination with Ⓛ UE movement. Pt. demonstrated poor motor control when reaching for objects and manipulating them. Pt.'s Ⓡ UE was observed to be flaccid. Pt. was observed repositioning Ⓡ UE when it fell off his lap. Pt. demonstrated ability to move his Ⓡ UE using the clasped hand method but was observed to wince in pain at movements beyond 90° of shoulder flexion. Pt. required max Ⓐ to support weight on Ⓡ UE while weight bearing when reaching positions.

A:      Pt. would benefit from activities that encourage dynamic balance to facilitate Ⓘ with dressing activity. Pt. would benefit from ADL training to improve Ⓡ UE weakness and incoordination of Ⓑ UEs. Pt. would benefit from scapular mobilization of Ⓡ UE to ↑ FROM.

P:      Pt. to be seen b.i.d. for 2 weeks to work on showering. Pt. will demonstrate ability to shower safely while standing with SBA in 2 weeks. Pt. will demonstrate ability to lather 80% of body with CGA in 1 week.

There are problems with the critical thinking involved in writing this note. In the "S" he reports that the patient is unable to communicate, then indicates in the "O" that the patient was able to communicate pain by wincing. It would be better to state in the "S" that the patient was unable to communicate verbally.

Secondly, the information is not categorized properly, with some assessment data occurring in the "O" section. For example:

*Pt. demonstrated ↓ ability to follow verbal instructions during tx. session.*
*Pt. demonstrated ↓ coordination with Ⓛ UE movement.*
*Pt. demonstrated poor motor control when reaching for objects and manipulating them.*

Third, there are some statements that sound good superficially but lack essential information, such as the following.

*Pt. was seen in the rehabilitation gym to increase functional movement.*

Functional movement of what? Or consider this statement (how many is multiple?):

*"...following multiple demonstrations."*

Fourth, the writer is inconsistent in the kinds of skills he hopes to see the patient develop. In the "A" section he suggests 2 weeks of treatment to independence in dressing. Then in the "P" section he sets a plan for showering. It would be better to use the same activity in both sections, even though the patient may be working on both.

Lastly, the writer does not really assess the data, probably because he has already included his assessment in his observation. He begins the assessment section with what the patient would benefit from.

The first thing that should be done to help this note is to move some pieces of information to the "A" and to add a statement about the impact it has on the patient's occupational performance. For example, rather than just moving the statement about decreased ability to follow verbal instructions to the "A," he might say:

*Pt.'s increased ability to follow verbal instructions during tx. session make multiple means of communication, such as tactile cues and demonstration, necessary. However, Ⓘ repositioning of Ⓡ UE when it fell off his w/c armrest indicates a good cognitive potential in rehab.*

When discussing decreased coordination, he might say:

*Pt.'s Ⓛ UE incoordination and Ⓡ UE flaccidity make a choice necessary between facilitating movement in the flaccid UE toward regaining function, or teaching compensatory skills and increasing coordination in uninvolved side.*

He also needs to assess some of his other findings, such as good sitting balance. He might say:

*Pt.'s stable static sitting balance indicates good potential for improvement of dynamic balance needed for ↑ Ⓘ in ADLs.*

This writer seems to have a good grasp of the principles of treatment, and a good ability to interpret his observations, but needs to work on organizing the material in his mind before beginning to write.

## Worksheet 12-10: The Almost Note

**What does this note need to make it better?**

S:      Pt. reports stiffness in hip Ⓛ, but improvement from previous pain. She states a preference for transferring to her left. Pt. states that she is willing to do "whatever it takes to get out of the hospital."

**O:**      Pt. seen in room for work on dressing and functional mobility.

     **Transfer:**      Pt. SBA for standing pivot transfer bed → w/c to the left

                        Pt. min Ⓐ with transfers w/c ⇆ toilet using grab bar

     **Mobility:**      Pt. SBA with VCs to flex trunk when rolling from supine to Ⓡ side

                        Pt. SBA supine → sit; min Ⓐ sit → stand

                        Pt. Ⓘ in w/c mobility

     **Dressing:**      Pt. Ⓘ in donning shirt

                        Pt. min Ⓐ with VCs to don bra while standing

                        Pt. Ⓘ in donning socks and shoes

                        Pt. min Ⓐ with walker and VC in donning underwear and pants

                        Pt. needs setup for dressing activities

     **UE ROM:**      Ⓛ UE—WFL

                        Ⓡ UE ↓ range in proximal shoulder flexion

     **Static standing:** Pt. CGA with walker Ⓑ UE support

     **Dynamic standing:** Pt. SBA with walker for balance

**A:**      Deficits noted in Ⓡ UE coordination, Ⓑ UE strength, and dynamic standing balance. Pt. Ⓘ in dressing EOB, but is min Ⓐ in dressing when standing with a walker. Ⓛ UE AROM is WFL but Ⓡ UE has deficits noted in shoulder flexion. Pt. needs SBA in bed mobility when rolling to unaffected side and min Ⓐ in sit → stand 2° ↓ UE strength. Pt. needs SBA for transfer to unaffected side in pivot transfer bed → w/c and min w/c ⇆ toilet. Pt. would benefit from skilled OT to continue UE strengthening and coordination exercises and to ↑ dynamic standing balance using walker, in order to ↑ Ⓘ in ADLs.

**P:**      Pt. to be seen b.i.d. for 30-minute sessions to continue to work on dynamic standing balance. Pt. will require SBA in grooming activities standing sink-side with standard walker within 2 weeks.

*Again, we have a note that seems good on the surface, but demonstrates some problems in critical thinking.*

*First, there is nothing in the "O" to show that skilled occupational therapy is being provided. The list of observations of assist levels fails to provide the richness of the treatment sessions. The therapist erroneously puts some of that information in the "A" section, rather than assessing her data.*

> *Pt. Ⓘ in dressing while sitting EOB, but is min Ⓐ in dressing when standing with a walker. Ⓛ UE AROM is WFL but Ⓡ UE has deficits noted in shoulder flexion. Pt. SBA in bed mobility when rolling to unaffected side and min Ⓐ in sit → stand 2° to ↓ UE strength. Pt. SBA for transfer to unaffected side in pivot transfer bed → w/c and min Ⓐ w/c ⇆ toilet.*

*Even in this expanded version, there is nothing to tell us what part of the task the assistance was for.*

*Second, the coordination deficits mentioned in the "A" section come out of the blue. There is no mention of coordination in the opening statement "...for work on dressing and functional mobility," nor is it mentioned in the "O." Thus the statement that coordination deficits are one of the problems noted and the statement that the patient would benefit from coordination exercises are unsubstantiated. Remember not to introduce any new information in the "A" section of your note.*

*Third, this therapist has used a non-standard abbreviation (VC) to mean "verbal cues". Since VC is a standard medical terminology for "vital capacity", it should not be used in this way.*

*The best thing for this therapist to do is to rewrite the "O" section, providing a more comprehensive picture of the treatment session. Then she needs to assess her data based on her observations. There needs to be an indication of how the observed data impacts the occupational performance of the patient, before the statements about what the patient would benefit from.*

*Depending on the assessment she makes, the plan to work on balance may be appropriate, or it may be only one of the things to be addressed.*

# NOTE TO THE READER

We invite your comments, criticisms, ideas, and suggestions for ways to make this book better or more useful to instructors, students, and beginning therapists. We also invite you to submit examples of documentation that you consider to be representative of some particular concept (such as conciseness). We are particularly interested in notes that represent "best practice" in occupational therapy today. If you work in an area of practice that you feel is under-represented, or if you have a note that you would like to see included, please send it to us for consideration in the next edition. We would also like to include more notes written by COTAs in the next edition, and would encourage COTAs to submit notes, so that the second edition will reflect more of the COTA influence in the profession.

When submitting a note, please include your name, address, and telephone number, along with your permission to publish the note. If your note is included in the next edition, you will receive full credit as author (or you may to choose to have an alias if you prefer). If you are teaching, please encourage your students to submit corrected copies of their best notes. Sometimes students think that their notes are not as good as those of practicing therapists, and this is not necessarily the case.

If you have ideas or comments on any of the topics presented here, or feel that documentation in your practice area is not thoroughly and accurately covered in this book, please let us hear from you. We would like to make this book reflective of all areas of practice, so that students graduate with exposure to documenting whatever area of OT practice they choose to enter.

Sherry Borcherding
c/o SLACK Incorporated
Professsional Book Division
6900 Grove Road
Thorofare, NJ 08086

# INDEX

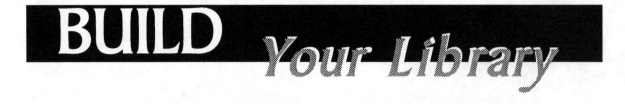

# BUILD *Your Library*